TEXTING THROUGH

Cancer

Ordinary Moments *of* Community, Love, *and* Healing

Jan Woodard

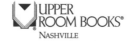

UPPER
ROOM BOOKS®
NASHVILLE

Library of Congress Cataloging-in-Publication Data

Names: Woodard, Jan, 1948–2020, author.

Title: Texting through cancer : ordinary moments of community, love, and healing / Jan Woodard. Description: Nashville, TN : Upper Room Books, 2021. | Includes bibliographical references. | Identifiers: LCCN 2020034276 (print) | LCCN 2020034277 (ebook) | ISBN 9780835819503 (hardcover) | ISBN 9780835819510 (mobi) | ISBN 9780835819527 (epub) Subjects: LCSH: Woodard, Jan, 1948–2020. | Breast—Cancer—Patients—Religious life. Classification: LCC BV4910.33 .W66 2021 (print) | LCC BV4910.33 (ebook) | DDC 248.8/619699449--dc23

LC record available at https://lccn.loc.gov/2020034276

LC ebook record available at https://lccn.loc.gov/2020034277

Printed in the United States of America

For Jim, who holds my heart.
We're two of the lucky ones.
All will be well, my love.

God quiets me with love.
—ZEPHANIAH 3:17, AP

CONTENTS

INTRODUCTION

All things came into being through him, and
without him not one thing came into being.
What has come into being in him was life,
and the life was the light of all people.

—JOHN 1:3-4

Leaves were beginning to bud across the chilly hills of central Pennsylvania a few years back when I drove to a silent retreat with total strangers in search of something, unsure what. Uncertainty is how spiritual adventures usually begin for me.

Knees to my chest, hair disheveled, my body wrapped in a blanket, I curled in a rocker most of the retreat and felt immersed in prayer as never before. Eight participants filled a small living room and prayed the scriptures every three hours for thirty-six hours with silence, walks, meals, and rest in between. Called the Liturgy of the Hours, we prayed through the life of Jesus, joining believers across the centuries since the time of Saint Benedict.

Out of this Benedictine practice of round-the-clock prayer, I discovered that somewhere on earth someone is always praying. Two years later, someone's prayer for people with cancer must have inspired a literary angel to plant a seed in my mind. It came almost like a dream as I tossed in bed, just days after breast cancer interrupted my life. I had requested prayer when I posted online that I was scheduled to have a biopsy, and friends flooded my inbox with words of encouragement that told me I was deeply loved. Somehow, I wanted to pass on their prayers, and my own faith, to others. *Why not ask the local newspaper editor if he'd like a column about this?* I thought. *It might help somebody.* Even the title came in that instant: "Texting Thru Cancer."

I phoned the newspaper editor the next morning before I could lose my nerve. He liked the idea. As I recovered from the heart-thumping shock of his "yes," he added, "It might help *you* too, writing your way through it." He nailed it. Writing a weekly column set my mind on others, prevented pity parties, and shifted my attention from fear to faith. I shared in my column and on my blog, janwoodard.com, messages that remind us we're never alone. I closed with *All will be well,* a phrase borrowed and adapted from Julian of Norwich. Her *Revelations of Divine Love,* written sometime in the late 1300s, is the oldest surviving book written by a woman in the English language.[1] I sometimes sputtered and tripped over her phrase, knowing personally how cancer ravages bodies, dreams, families, and lives. But deeper still lay the confidence that *God is with us*—redeeming and transforming suffering into something sacred and life-giving.

Julian's statement of faith reminds me to rest, breathe, and sink into God's goodness. I invite you to do just that as you read this book. A dozen faith disciplines are interspersed throughout, with suggestions on how to embrace them as your own. A year before my cancer was detected, I went on a Celtic Christian pilgrimage as part of a spiritual formation program I was participating in. This experience deeply influenced my spirituality and intimacy with God, Jesus, and the Holy Spirit—the Sacred Three—and is a cornerstone of this book.

If you find a connection within these pages, it means we breathe the same air. Everybody faces challenging times. Maybe it's not cancer, but life throws obstacles at anyone with a heartbeat.

Even you. Simply because you're human.

Thank you to those people on their knees right now, wearing down the carpet, praying for people with cancer. It makes a difference. Things don't always end happily ever after on this side of eternity, but your prayers are like lampposts, lighting the path so others don't stumble in the dark.

Whoever you are, we're companions on this bumpy pilgrimage.

All will be well,

Jan Woodard
January 2020

A WORD ABOUT FAITH PRACTICES

"Abide in me as I abide in you. Just as the branch cannot bear fruit by itself unless it abides in the vine, neither can you unless you abide in me."

—JOHN 15:4

Faith practices keep us centered on our spiritual journey, guiding us like painted lines on a highway. As the phrase suggests, they take practice, like learning to drive. Also called disciplines, the practices found in this book strengthen my faith for the hard times, helping me to abide in the love of Jesus. They equip me to survive one day at a time with this disease, knowing I'm encircled spiritually by others who practice them as well. Picture a rainbow—the beauty we see results from its range of hues, melding together. The abundant Christian life is like that, blending believers with a variety of spiritual practices that enrich us all as we bow before God Most High. My prayer is that you sense yourself being drawn near to God through the indwelling Holy Spirit while reading this book. Some of the suggested practices may fit you and your schedule better than others. Some are best done in solitude; others apply to our life together in beloved community.

BEGINNINGS

Do not fear, for I am with you,
do not be afraid, for I am your God;
I will strengthen you, I will help you,
I will uphold you with my victorious right hand.

—ISAIAH 41:10

I found the lump myself. Just before bed, I fingered something foreign under my T-shirt. Hard as a dried pea, near my armpit. How could *that* be anything? I asked my husband, Jim, fresh from a shower, to feel it.

"Better get it checked out," he said, pulling me into his warmth.

I scribbled a note on my nightstand to call for a mammogram in the morning but then ignored it. I hate how that mammogram machine clamps my breast like an angry alligator. Was that only an excuse? Winter drifted into spring. Sweat from my water glass eventually faded the ink.

If only cancer disappeared as easily.

In early April, fear chilled me awake one night. The next morning, I went to the hospital's women's center and discovered they had an immediate opening. Once properly gowned, I said to the technician, "Let's do this!", hoping my good attitude would reap good results.

Isn't that how it's supposed to work?

Sounding cautious, my doctor telephoned that evening to say I needed to follow up on my mammogram with an ultrasound the next day. Soon enough, I was in a darkened room with another technician, who glided a warm wand across my breast.

"Yes," he nodded toward a screen. "There's a tumor. It looks like cancer, but you'll need a biopsy to confirm." Jim entered the room and plied the poor guy with questions, as if information would make a difference. My mind was numb, my face wet with tears. After a week that felt like forever, I was back for the biopsy, praying any nasty cells were neatly contained, as easy to remove as several harmless cysts had been decades earlier. I'd get good news and celebrate with a quick prayer of thanks and a hike in the park.

In the middle of the procedure the surgeon said, "Let's sample this lymph node. It looks suspicious."

Instantly, my world changed. I wanted to jump off the table and tear out of the room. Sue, the nurse by my side, clasped my hand, reading my fear as I squeezed hers. Not only surgery but chemotherapy and radiation—cancer's trifecta—now loomed over me like a tornado, sucking my breath away.

Jim and I sat at the supper table that evening, unable to swallow a bite. He asked a blessing, holding my hand. Opening his eyes, he looked into mine and said, "I won't let you go. If I have to hold onto your feet to keep you from going, I will." I tried to smile at the image, but it wouldn't come, as if life and death were playing tug of war and I was the prize.

Will I lose my hair?

Will I lose my breast?

Will I lose my life?

Over the next twelve months a breast was cut off, my hair fell out, and my eyebrows vanished. But as my body grew fragile from treatments, my inner life flourished. Cancer waltzed into our lives like an unwanted dance partner, but it didn't get to choose the music. Through texts, Facebook posts, emails, cards, and responses to my newspaper column, hundreds of friends walked alongside Jim and me on this unexpected journey.

> *I'll be praying for you, dear lady.*
>
> *You're on my heart! I stand with you.*
>
> *God will be your guide and strength.*

From the start, I was never alone. If I ever doubted the value of family, friends, and my faith community, I never will again.

A beginning, not an end.

All will be well.

GRACE FROM
THE GET-GO

[The Lord] said to me, "My grace is sufficient for
you, for my power is made perfect in weakness."
Therefore I will boast all the more gladly about my
weaknesses, so that Christ's power may rest on me.

—2 CORINTHIANS 12:9, NIV

My first newspaper column, "Texting Thru Cancer," began with
these texts:

> **Me:** *Ultrasound of lump today. Doc is highly
> suspicious it's cancer. He said we're early in the
> game.*
>
> **Big Sis Carol:** *This is a scary time for you.
> Remembering you with love & prayers.*

My mind and emotions were all over the place. At times I was
a total mess, planning my funeral. The next moment I breathed
deeply and pictured myself in an auditorium at my grandson
Eli's high school graduation. He's only five years old.

This was new terrain for me, but I knew I was not alone.
My twin sister, Marilyn, a pastoral counselor, called the moment
after my text appeared on her phone. I heard heartache in her
voice, tighter than usual, when she told me I'm entering "the

fellowship of suffering." This is the crazy, upside-down idea that through suffering we identify with the suffering of others and can be there to comfort one another as God comforts us. Not a club I'd choose to join but a circle of intimacy with those who understand the struggle.

Because attitude and prayer change things in ways we'll never comprehend, I decided to overcome fears that stalked my mind by exposing them to light. I announced my upcoming biopsy on Facebook with this post: "If you're a positive person who prays, please join me in thanking God that love wins!" Messages of hope lit up my screen, hundreds of them. Feeling bubble wrapped in prayer, I underwent that test. A few days later, Jim and I sat in an exam room. The surgeon shook my hand and started examining my breasts. His silence dialed up my foreboding.

"What did they find?" I finally asked.

"You have cancer," he said, and continued my exam as calmly as if he had just said I had an ingrown toenail.

Jim groaned. Visions of his dad's final days fighting colon cancer crossed my mind, but something within me hardened into stony determination—I will survive this.

Still feeling bubble wrapped, I sent a group text the minute Jim and I walked outside.

> **Me:** Biopsy shows breast cancer cells. All will be well.
>
> **Nephew:** With each breath, know you are loved and you love in return.
>
> **Daughter:** I love you, Mama.
>
> **Friend:** I so want to jump through this cell phone and hug you, sweet lady!

With the car already packed, Jim and I zipped out of town to spend the weekend with our daughters. Before we left, we paused in the women's center, where Donna, an RN, hugged me tight. Her eyes brimmed, and then she suggested we write down what we were thankful for as we drove across Pennsylvania. Another audacious, upside-down notion. We did it without much heart, at first. Yet the list kept growing: family, friends, modern medicine, Chewbacca (our dog), Yellow Creek Lake, blooming redbuds, mountains dressed in spring green, and a road to carry us from here to there and home again.

A PET scan showed the cancer was localized. This was good news, but still I asked myself, *Is this really happening?* I felt like I was losing control of everything, but stubborn faith told me something good would come out of this.

> **Breast cancer survivor:** *For whatever reason, and we may never know, I feel strongly that this is God's grace, and I don't know why, but in some way, it is a gift.*

I knew, even then, that grace would carry me.

All will be well.

The Practice of Gratitude

Rejoice in the Lord always; again I will say,
rejoice!... Do not be anxious about anything,
but in everything by prayer and pleading
with thanksgiving let your requests be made
known to God. And the peace of God, which
surpasses all comprehension, will guard
your hearts and minds in Christ Jesus.

—PHILIPPIANS 4:4, 6-7, NASB (EMPHASIS ADDED)

I discovered the spiritual practice of being thankful early in my Christian walk. After my husband suffered burns in a kitchen fire in 1973, my Bible teacher lent me a dog-eared paperback of *Prison to Praise* by Merlin R. Carothers. I'd never heard the concept of being grateful for *everything* before that, but then I noticed Paul says, "Rejoice in the Lord always; again I will say, rejoice!" (Phil. 4:4, NASB). Paul wrote and suffered in a Roman prison and knew how hard it was to choose to be thankful, no matter what.

For me, "no matter what" includes living with cancer. When I praise and thank God in the midst of my circumstances, they may not change, but I do. My husband committed his life to Jesus because of our fire. At the same time, I learned what it means to be a Spirit-led believer, depending upon the Trinity to help me live with courage and gratitude.

It was divine timing when a nurse suggested Jim and I look for signposts of God's goodness the same day my diagnosis of breast cancer was confirmed. We discovered that our gratitude list began to grow when we changed our focus.

* * *

Some people enjoy creating a list of things they are thankful for as a way to end their day. Before bed, list five experiences or encounters for which you are grateful. It might be a friend who came to your mind during the day, a scripture you read that held a special message for you, or the fresh vegetables from your garden you enjoyed for lunch. The more challenging your circumstances, the more these recollections might mean to you. Record your list in a journal so you can return to it again and again.

LETTING GO

When we were children,
we thought and reasoned
as children do.
But when we grew up,
we quit our childish ways.
Now all we can see of God
is like a cloudy picture
in a mirror.
Later we will see him
face to face.
We don't know everything,
but then we will,
just as God completely
understands us.

—1 CORINTHIANS 13:11-12, CEV

Tara, my oldest daughter, and her family are moving to New Zealand. *The other side of the world.* My voice quivers only slightly when I say it. New Zealand is not California or Florida—places I can reach by plane in a few hours. My heart aches. The South Pacific is a long stretch from the low, mined-out hills of western Pennsylvania where I live, and I like my grandchildren within arm's reach. I try to picture Tara's boys having grand adventures but swallow hard as questions swirl: How fast will they grow up? Will they remember I love them? When will we see one another again?

When I heard there was a tumor growing in my breast, my grief turned to steely resolve. Our boys *will* have a grandma living in this three-story house when they return. (They call me "Tall House Grandma.") What seems right now like distant goals ease my anguish—heal well enough to travel, wrap my family in hugs, kayak a fiord, and meet some Kiwis (New Zealanders). Good reasons to hope and heal. At least they don't have to see me sick.

Meanwhile, I set out tables for a neighborhood yard sale, craving mental and physical space for what lies ahead and wondering how I'll survive cancer when I can't even organize a bookshelf. While it's good to get rid of stuff, there's one thing I don't relinquish as easily as books and dishes.

> **Me:** *After forty-six years, I had my wedding ring cut off.*
>
> **Daughter Julie:** *Oh, Mom.*

Jim slipped that ring on my hand at the altar in 1969, and I never took it off. Because my knuckle is now thicker than my little band of gold, it had to go. After a jeweler clipped it, my friend Faye consoled me with biscotti at a local bakery. "We can either think things happen *to* us or *for* us," she said. I choose to think the latter.

***

Something in my great-niece's pink face resembles my Grandma Watrous. Brushing my cheek against Maria's, I kissed her hair and held her close. She tried to nuzzle against something that wasn't there before deciding my tightly wrapped torso wasn't anything like her mama's.

Marilyn and I gave our bluebird china tea set, the one we had used as children, to Maria as a baptismal gift, packaged in the original red and blue box and stamped with the price—$3.98. Mother and Daddy hid it for us under the Christmas tree when we were about six. Mom fringed the blue gingham napkins and tablecloth for a miniature maple table, and we served each other tea while seated in the alcove of our Cape Cod bedroom, two scoops of sugar in each miniature cup.

My own daughters wore big, brimmed hats for their tea parties, pretending to be grown-ups. As adults, we look back and wish we could recapture those times. Infants, though, live entirely in the moment. Holding a baby is reassuring, a way of touching other generations. On one of my last visits with Grandma Watrous (Maria's great-great grandmother), she gave me a box of family photos. In it was a postcard from the 1800s of a sprawling family posing on a country porch. There's a tiny swatch of auburn hair attached, the same shade as Julie's. Perhaps it was a birth announcement never mailed, tucked away in a desk for a century or more. A reader of my blog suggested maybe it was a death notice from an age when children often didn't survive.

When I offered my girls, all grown up, a clipping of their own baby hair, one chose to keep it and the other shook her head and said no thanks. I winced to see those curls go in the wastebasket. Curl by curl, a handful of childhood history now gone.

I pondered all this as Brenda, my hairdresser, was about to bob my locks (think Dorothy Hamill 2.0). I stopped coloring my hair after my diagnosis and since then gray roots have sprouted like weeds in my untended garden. Will I lose it all?

A breast cancer survivor told me her hair started falling out shortly after beginning chemotherapy. She had her head shaved after that and scattered the clippings in her yard. Later she found birds gathering bits to weave in their nests. With that image she passed along tender courage of how all things work together for good in God's mysterious ways. I am reminded that beauty is found in every age and stage.

Another friend texted a verse I've prayed in the past for my kids but for some reason had laid aside. Reading it, I felt my backbone growing stronger: "being confident of this, that he who began a good work in you will carry it on to completion until the day of Christ Jesus" (Phil. 1:6, NIV). When fear threatens to undo me, subtly drawing me to darker places, praying God's Word becomes my nesting hideaway.

There is a time for everything. Now is a time for letting go—of books, rings, tea sets, hair, and wanting to be someone other than who I am. In its place is an inner knowing that I'm exactly who and where I'm meant to be.

A high school friend serving in campus ministry: I'm so privileged to be part of your journey! Be anxious for NOTHING, but in EVERYTHING be thankful.

Me: Amen!

All will be well.

WAITING ROOM

Don't be afraid or dismayed.
I, your God, am with you.
I've got this. My hand will be in yours.

—ISAIAH 41:10, 13, AP

I choke on the words, "I have cancer."

I can't—I won't—say them.

I won't allow it to define me.

Cancer interrupts everything. Swamps me in anxieties that snake out of the murky darkness. But here's the thing—it also makes each moment and every person more precious. And there is good news. Friends and I exchange posts after the PET scan reveals that cancer cells are limited to one quadrant of my chest. Hooray!

> **Friend:** Words cannot describe the relief your message brings. Tough times ahead for sure but HOPE.
>
> **Me:** More tests scheduled. Please pray they don't find more lymph nodes with nasty cells present.
>
> **Friend:** God is near in our lowest times. God is holding your hand and saying, "I love you, my child."

I feel cocooned in that love as I sit in God's waiting room. Waiting for test results. Waiting for surgery. Waiting for a treatment plan. While I wait, I compile a list on a yellow pad of people who have survived cancer. It's long and growing daily.

Also cocooning me as I wait is the love of a Kenyan family that relocated to Pennsylvania years ago. Embracing them as our own is one of my family's great blessings. It is my honor to have Elizabeth and Rafael call me "Mama" and their children, Fiona, Melody, and Josiah, to think of me as a grandmother. One day Elizabeth sends this text from Yale, where she is studying:

> *Yale International Student Fellowship and the Women's Bible Study at Trinity Church will fast and pray for you all week, Mama. Victory is on your side.*

Waiting is hard, yes. Saying goodbye to my sweeties traveling a world away is harder still. When my heart ponders, asking *How can this be happening?* I hear God whisper to me, *Don't be afraid.* And a quiet peace reminds me God has this.

All will be well.

MASTECTOMY DAY JOURNAL

Whoever dwells in the shelter of the Most High
will rest in the shadow of the Almighty.

—PSALM 91:1, NIV

7:00 a.m.	They said arrive at seven, surgery at nine. The receptionist hands me a card made by a nighttime staffer, who happens to be a member of a women's group I lead at church. I grip it like a life preserver with eyes blurred, thinking how insane all this is. Maybe somebody made a mistake. Maybe they'll cancel.
8:00 a.m.	People stream into my room. Pastor Kathy prays and holds my hand. Donna from the women's center brings me a handmade bag in autumn colors. My colors. Inside I find a quilt, a "knitty titty" (small but still too big for my petite bosom), and a corset with pockets for drains from my side. She smiles with a look that says, "Be brave." I feel anything but.
8:30 a.m.	Our son, Brett, wanders in and out with his camera, looking lost, just like Jim and I do. Within an hour there's a pathetic picture on Facebook—me in bed, smiling, eyes closed, an IV in my arm. Later I learn

it activated an army of prayer warriors. My bubble wrap is holding its own.

10:00 a.m. No surgery yet. My friend Linda keeps vigil nearby in the crowded waiting room, praying. I never see her but sense the warmth of her kindness. "I felt I was supposed to be there," she says later.

12:00 p.m. I wait and wait. The surgeon stops in and apologizes. Emergencies delayed my turn on the table. Yes, it's the left breast we're removing. And, yes, I'm going home this evening, thank you very much. Who wants to hang around a hospital after they slice off a body part! He initials my left arm with a red marker.

1:00 p.m. Jim's lips brush my face, and with that lost puppy look he whispers, "I love you." I'm rolled down the hall.

* * *

Later: I feel like a mummy, my torso tightly wrapped in wide bandages, with two drainage tubes dangling. Struggling to breathe, I'm in a timeless fog. My fingers wander to my chest. It's gone. Jim folds my hand in his. *How's he feeling about this?* I wonder. I doze. Our girls arrive in the evening from Princeton and Philadelphia, surrounding me in family-ness. After eleven, I'm wheeled to our car.

12:00 a.m. Home. Julie enters my darkened bedroom with a vial of lavender oil. "This will help you sleep," she says, rubbing a cool drop on my forehead. Before drifting off, I realize it's the first time in sixteen years our nuclear family of five has been alone under our tall roof. I almost cry but instead fall asleep.

***

In the following days, I'm embraced in the colors and flavors of love. Kenyan children bring sunflowers. Palestinian neighbors carry in tabbouleh. Church folks schedule meals for weeks. A lady with a green thumb and a pink hat plants a prayer garden in her yard in my honor.

Tara hugs me long and hard and then heads home to pack for her family's move to New Zealand. My legs wobble.

"I'll see you on the other side," she says, then laughs. "Of the world, that is."

These things, not cancer, bring me to tears.

In my autumn-colored bag is a DVD advising lifelong exercises "to maintain a full range of motion." Like that's going to happen. Okay, with the kids gone, I may do a few steps if a song calls my name and maybe some stretches. Since I'm a dance school dropout and resist exercise, it will definitely be for an audience of one.

Years ago, Tara introduced me to *The Wounded Healer* by Henri J. M. Nouwen. I am reminded that we're all somewhere on the brokenness spectrum. It's okay to admit I'm undone by all of this—the fear, the love, the prayers, the thought of that unspeakable word, *cancer*.

A teacher in Ohio whose family just traveled through its own cancer scare messages me:

> *I know how precious it is to walk through a challenge with the unshakable assurance that Jesus is holding you. Thank you, Lord, that*

there is nothing about Jan's situation that
catches you by surprise. Do what you do—bring
your healing ... peace ... joy ... wisdom.

I drink in this prayer. If I end up going through chemo, I may be out of the sun this summer, but I will never be beyond God's care.

Fellow breast cancer survivor Natalie Glaser journaled through her treatments and honed her thoughts into in a book that blesses others, *Don't Call Me Brave–I Was Not Alone.* Natalie and I became friends after meeting at another writer's book signing. She messages me:

I journal a prayer most mornings. If only for
a brief moment, I hear God talking to me.
Journaling can be personal and vulnerable but
so inspiring to others. Thanks for writing your
words so that I could hear God invite me to
take more time to write.

All will be well.

The Practice of Journaling

My tongue is the pen of a skillful writer.

—PSALM 45:1, NIV

Journaling is simply writing in a notebook or diary, usually for the writer's eyes only. The root of both *journal* and *journey* is the French word *jour,* meaning "day," so think of a journal as recording travels through events, thoughts, and spiritual responses that comprise our days. We don't have to journal every day for it to strengthen our spiritual lives, but the more faithful we are to this—and all spiritual disciplines—the more it adds depth to our experience. And although a journal is a private space to work through thoughts, our journals can inspire others. I have my grandmother's diary, as she would have called it, from her visit to her brother's grave in France following World War I. It's a precious family record written in fading pencil in a small paper notebook.

There are no rules for journaling. Don't worry about writing complete sentences or using proper grammar. The only thing I do consistently is write the date, weather or temperature, and my location if I'm away from home at the top of the page. I find it easiest to write in a spiral-bound journal that lies flat, but you might prefer a different kind. Sometimes I use colored pencils to add drawings. When I journal on paper with pen in hand, I experience an intimacy that I missed the few times I tried journaling with a keyboard and screen. I'm usually talking to God when I journal, putting my prayers onto paper, honestly pouring out my feelings to the Almighty One who best knows me, which may be why one of my spiritual mentors says journaling is his most meaningful discipline. Letter writing can be another form of journaling, intended to be read by one or more recipients, so we might think of Paul's New Testament letters as journaling inspired by God.

A friend tells me she believes writing strengthens our connection to God. Think about this in terms of journaling. Our writing connects us to God, the greatest Spirit who gives us understanding for every struggle and hurdle. I pray for you—and every person dealing with diseases—that you find this connection and know God is in control. I have always believed when we write, our souls communicate with God, and the exchange itself is healing. May the words you write become food for your soul.

* * *

Find a spot in your home where you can journal easily, with a comfortable place to sit and your supplies at hand. Maybe beside the window in your house that affords you the best view of the outdoors. Set aside time to spend with pen and paper, writing God a letter each day for twenty-one days. See what happens. Do you feel closer to God? Does it become easier for you to unburden yourself while writing? to catalog your joys? Apart from your intentional journaling time, don't limit yourself to that one space. Keep a small notebook or some index cards in your purse so you can jot down your thoughts during the day, wherever you are. (Some people enjoy using a cell phone app for this purpose.) You never know when God might want a word with you, a word worth capturing.

THIN PLACES

God saw all that he had made,
and it was very good.

—GENESIS 1:31, NIV

I watched the moon rise over a tree-lined ridge in County Wicklow, Ireland, and later hopscotched by ferries to Iona, a tiny island off Scotland's coast.

"You never know what the future might hold," I said to myself years ago, before I had the opportunity to take a Celtic Christian pilgrimage in 2015 as part of the spiritual formation program in which I'm enrolled at Pittsburgh Theological Seminary. As the years pass, I often revisit those ancient sites in my mind.

Did something nudge me to go? I believe that God was preparing me in ways I didn't understand for a future I didn't expect.

The journey introduced me to believers from the first centuries of the Christian faith. In class discussions I learned Celtic Christianity is a way of looking at the world that celebrates the goodness and grace of the Sacred Three, the Trinity. It sees a God of wonder and proposes God's love as our strong tower—like the ancient stone towers I touched in Ireland. Along the way, I discovered "thin places," as the Celts call them, where the veil between heaven and earth seems translucent. On my first night in Dublin, the pilgrimage director, Rebecca Cole-Turner, told the group about encircling prayers. This is a distinctively Celtic way of coming before the Sacred Three called a *caim,* Gaelic for "protection," enfolding those praying and those prayed for in God's secure love by drawing a circle—real or imaginary—around all involved. On my knees on a cross-stitched kneeler in St. Patrick's Cathedral in Dublin, I felt encompassed by God's angels, guarding and guiding me.

Saint Patrick set the pattern for those who followed the new faith he introduced. His band of men sought God's protection, singing boldly as they tramped through enemy territory. I sometimes feel that's where I am in this fight with cancer—in enemy territory. "To know that Christ stands behind us is to know that, in an ultimate way, we are safe," writes Marilyn Chandler McEntyre in *Christ, My Companion: Meditations on the Prayer of St. Patrick*.[2] She added this, a few pages later, "Wherever you go, God got there first and is waiting for you."[3]

I sensed that on the isles, and I know it now.

The power of memory transports me from my present hard place to rocky Iona, a Scottish thin place. While others took a strenuous hike one morning, I chose a solitary one, accompanied by inquisitive sheep. Reaching a gate in the meadow above the sea, I left my companions behind and skittered down a path to the rocks and waves, in need of quiet time with God. On my return, I leaned heavily on my walking stick, pressing into fierce gusts, eyes shielded by my rain jacket's flapping hood, with nary an islander in sight. I imagine that if any of the young folks employed on the island spotted my bent figure, they shrugged me off as another zany crone treading this sacred isle. Warm soup and friendly faces welcomed me for a late lunch. Looking back, I know the windy breath of God's Spirit strengthened me that morning for the unknowns of today. Later, in the lingering light of a June evening in the North Atlantic, I sat in the chill of the great stone abbey, joining sixteen hundred years of pilgrims seeking and praising God on that renowned bit of land.

Cancer helps me turn ordinary moments—laughing, weeping, eating, worshiping, writing, gardening, praying, discovering—into encircling acts of holy protection. And humbling moments too, such as leaning on my husband and others like I did on my walking stick in Iona. I have learned from both sides of the Atlantic that any place can be a thin place. I don't have to cross an ocean or step into the past to find signs of God's Spirit breaking through.

The morning after my mastectomy, a text from Marilyn offered yet another such sign:

> *I asked Mom to send you a cardinal this morning.*

Within minutes a bright-red fellow perched on our deck feeder. He and his mate have chirped there ever since. My registered nurse buddy Sue, who clasped my hand during that awful biopsy, said she felt from the beginning I'd see signs of the Lord's presence throughout the adversities of cancer.

I know my healing begins where I'm planted and that God is only a breath away.

All will be well.

PRAYER SOCKS

"By the tender mercy of our God,
the dawn from on high will break upon us,
to give light to those who sit in darkness
and in the shadow of death,
to guide our feet into the way of peace."

—LUKE 1:78-79

At first, I planned to skip past chemotherapy, as if staying alive might be as easy as skipping over jail on a Monopoly board. Statistics scribbled on a board by an oncologist indicated that chemotherapy would only minimally improve my chances of surviving breast cancer. That made my decision easy: I'd go straight to radiation after recovering from my mastectomy. Hey, maybe I could even skip that! Why suffer through treatments for little or nothing in return?

Then Jim and I happened by our church sanctuary one evening where E. K. Gardner, a nursing professor and saxophone player, waited for the worship team to arrive for practice. When we asked his advice, he motioned for us to sit with him on a pew. "God will show you what to do," he said quietly, almost like a prayer. "God will give you peace, and you'll know."

But doubt, not peace, darkened my mind. My physicians all agreed that because of the aggressiveness of the cancer cells, my best option was to smack 'em hard with everything on the shelf, even if the statistics did not seem not all that promising. A physician's assistant at Magee Women's Hospital eased my concern after the surgery, however, when she said, "We consider you healed. This is all prevention!"

Healed. I liked how that sounded. I wanted to stop there, but I could not shut out the part about prevention. Surgery should have dug out all the cancer, but let's lower the chances of bad cells ever showing up again. Was I really saying yes to six months of chemo?

It felt unreal, like I was watching a movie about somebody else. But as soon as I decided to proceed with chemo, peace came. I slept; I smiled. I did, however, sputter and choke on the idea at the last minute. The night before another surgery (to insert a port under my skin for injections), I fidgeted my fingers nervously, as if plotting to run away when I knew there was no escape. Jim beckoned me to his arms and prayed, "Encourage and protect my wife, Lord. Be her peace. We trust this to you."

Have I mentioned how much I love this man? His prayer settled me. I messaged Lynette, an ovarian cancer patient, on Facebook:

> *I'll get a port tomorrow and then begin chemo*
> *... you know what this is like.*
>
> **Lynette:** *Cancer really is life changing. You're in my prayers! The port is the best thing I've ever done; it makes everything easier.*

As I awaited surgery, I journaled in a hospital bed, wearing a gift of psychedelic-colored socks to keep my feet warm. Later I posted:

Home from surgery, everything's fine. Feeling blessed by your prayers, love . . . more than I can take in . . . wearing prayer socks from a friend. My feet were covered in prayer . . . and the rest of me.

Spiritual formation classmate: *Know we're praying for you at First Presbyterian in Pasadena, Texas.*

Church small-group friend: *You are so often on my heart. Love and prayers.*

Cousin and thyroid cancer survivor: *Praying constantly!*

Former student, also recovering from breast cancer: *I think of you every day. Take care.*

Sender of prayer socks: *Love you!*

Brain cancer patient: *I have a pair of socks knit by a friend. I didn't think to call them prayer socks, but I bet they were prayed over by my friend as she knit them. You're covered toe to head! Blessings on that port. May all that goes through it bring healing.*

Chemo comes with risks and benefits. I'm more than a percentage on a computer screen—I'm a woman who knows my source of strength and wholeness. A girlfriend's text said it best:

God has this!

All will be well.

NOW FAITH

My times are in your hands.

—PSALM 31:15, NIV

Some moments change us forever. Moving to an unfamiliar place, like my daughter Tara's family. Finding a lump in your breast. We can't control some things, but we can choose how we approach the mountains and valleys of our lives that divide the now and forever.

The evening of my breast biopsy, Sue, my registered nurse friend who held my hand earlier in the day, gave me a gift when we met for prayer group. It meant even more when she said she received it from the first woman she mentored through breast cancer. The small mirror, inscribed with "One Day at a Time," sits on my kitchen windowsill.

One nanosecond is more like it. Oh, sweet Jesus, help me through this one.

Hearing that cancer had migrated to at least one lymph node sent me into a wilderness. This was before my PET scan, when a Mt. Everest-sized question overshadowed me: How far have those crappy cancer cells traveled? Lab results showed cancer in two of fourteen lymph nodes removed from my armpit. While I was trying to take that in, the oncologist mentioned another concern. Simply put, one cancerous node resembled a baggie with a broken seal, meaning cancer cells could spill out and spread farther.

Where is my faith when I need it? I thought of the tiny globe on a gold chain in my jewel box, a mustard seed inside. A gift from Grandma Watrous. That's what I need, I told myself, faith like Grandma's. A mustard seed of stuff powerful enough to move this mountain.

Tears spilled maddeningly as I adjusted to the new reports. I wore sunglasses a lot. Of course, I took them off the day my hairdresser, Brenda, trimmed my shoulder-length, brunette-from-a-bottle hair, preparing me for the day when my hair might be missing altogether. I glanced at my reflection before she picked up her scissors.

I wasn't sixteen, or even sixty, but I still missed my hair.

Hebrews 11 begins, "Now, faith is. . . ." Brenda, whose mother has Alzheimer's disease, caught my attention when she said she depends on "now faith" to carry her through every hour of every day. "Encourage one another every day, as long as it is *still* called 'today'" says Hebrews 3:13 (NASB).

And it's always just that—it's never yesterday or tomorrow—it's always today.

Unless, of course, it isn't.

I messaged Tara in New Zealand (seventeen hours ahead of us, with opposite seasons):

> *I'm trying to grasp that our today is your yesterday, and our tomorrow is your today. Time is upside down by clock and season. It's still light here at almost 9:00 p.m. I've just cleared the table from a late supper, and it should be lunchtime tomorrow there. The one constant is love. And dishes.*

Tara was born at dawn on the summer solstice. We celebrated her birthday on the longest, brightest day of the year, June 21. In New Zealand, it arrives on the shortest and darkest. All this to say that time is relative. In the midst of forever, what we have is now.

On Father's Day I relaxed in my Steelers chair on Jim's fishing boat after kayaking the tree-lined edge of Yellow Creek Lake. It was evening, our first time on the water since my mastectomy six weeks earlier. A full moon appeared on a pink horizon and rose over the lake like a luminous pearl, while a fiery sunset reflected in the waters lapping the opposite shore. We had to turn our heads to drink in the radiance of both, letting go of one in order to enjoy the other.

As I released images of yesterday in order to face today, a stirring of memories remained, empowering me with God's help to move forward. Chemotherapy begins Thursday.

One day at a time, sweet Jesus.

All will be well.

PINPOINTS OF LIGHT

"Believe in the light while you have the light,
so that you may become children of light."

—JOHN 12:36, NIV

Me: Going to a healing service in Grove City.

Neighbor: Praying it's what you hope it will be.

A month after my surgery, Jim and I walked hand-in-hand across the tree-lined campus of Grove City College toward the entrance of a towering stone chapel. Before stepping inside, he asked what I hoped would happen that evening. I didn't have a clue, but with chemo about to begin I felt an urgency to be there. Did I expect healing to flow? Hopefully. To sense God's Spirit moving? Definitely.

Powerful worship welcomes the Trinity's presence. I felt the company of heaven in that arched stone chapel like I did in St. Patrick's Cathedral a year earlier. I smiled at the opening song, Chris Tomlin's "Good Good Father." This was the third time at consecutive services that the same song kicked off worship. It seemed the Spirit wanted to make sure Jim and I got the memo—we're God's beloved kids, and that's that. On the way home, I texted:

We absolutely were supposed to be there.

Neighbor: Never doubted that for a minute!

The apostle John, who knew Jesus intimately, wrote, "in him was life, and the life was the light of all people. The light shines in the darkness, and the darkness did not overcome it" (John 1:4-5). Light overpowers darkness, every time. I left that service feeling like somebody had switched on the lights. When fear creeps in on dark nights, I need to reach for my flashlight and shine it on that verse.

We all know people struggling with a life-threatening crisis or disease. There are no easy, pie-in-the-sky answers. I'm learning to trust that Jesus is with us in our suffering, and God somehow uses the unthinkable to mold us into the image of his suffering Son. Ilga, a faithful friend of mine, was widowed while still young. She wrote to me out of deep wisdom and deep loss:

> *God never wastes anything. We're always praying God will keep us out of deep waters or the fiery furnace, but oh, the eternal blessings that come out of them!*

God doesn't cause disease, accidents, or acts of terror. But if we allow it, our grieving God gathers up our broken pieces, like shards of stained glass, and creates something of beauty that light can shine through. It takes courage and prayers to hold this fragile world together. I'd like to see a worldwide prayer rally, a revival of hope. It won't begin in a stadium or cathedral. Instead, world-changing, light-generating prayer starts with the individual and moves on to where two or three of us come together on our knees.

I once saw a photo of Ireland from space that showed pinpoints of light glowing across the island. From God's perspective, perhaps our prayer gatherings are like that—points of light shining hope into a dark world. "For where two or three are gathered in my name, I am there among them" (Matt. 18:20).

All will be well.

The Practice of Worship

You are the LORD Most High over all the earth;
You are exalted far above all gods.

—PSALM 97:9, NASB

We don't always think of worship as an intentional discipline because it's just what Christians do, right? If we could ask the angels what comprises worship, they'd probably say people have yet to glimpse a spark of the glories of worshiping our Redeemer—and how could we on this side of heaven?

We can worship anywhere, alone or with others. I treasure both my solitude with the Lord and worshiping in community. I don't always feel like going to church on Sunday, but it's my practice, regardless of how I feel. As long as I'm healthy enough to be around other people, I'll be there. When I'm not, I can honor the sabbath and Yahweh by recognizing the Spirit's presence where I am, hearing my Creator's voice in everything. The song of a small Carolina wren at my bird feeder is praise equal to the "Hallelujah Chorus" if, as I'm listening, I lift my soul to the Sacred Three.

Worship increases intimacy with Immanuel, God with Us, and leads naturally into the messy business of loving other people. Pastor Eric Park, a longtime friend, challenged his Facebook friends to think of worship in terms of surrender, asking, "What portion of my life did I yield to the Lordship of Jesus today?"

followed by, "How much of myself did I dare to place upon the altar of God's grace?"

Worship isn't something we select from a cafeteria line of faith practices. We're created for it. We might not always realize it, but our souls yearn for it.

* * *

Worship begins with an attitude of the heart, bowing low in confession and adoration before the mysteries of God, and then carrying that wonder within, a flame that draws others to its warmth and light. To enter into a spirit of worship, breathe deeply and let one of the Trinity's names speak to you. (I often use the Lord Most High to lift my soul in praise.) Imagine yourself intentionally approaching Jesus with a surrendered heart, not as a servant but as a beloved child. Offer up your praise, petition, intercession, and confession to God, all the while remaining open to whatever the time of worship has in store for you. If you're not able to worship in community, develop some rituals that you can use to mark your intention at home. Consider including some of the more formal elements of traditional worship, such as singing hymns and reading scripture.

THE REST OF MY LIFE

"Come to me, everyone tired with heavy
burdens, and I will give you rest."

—MATTHEW 11:28, AP

I find a shiny bracelet dangling on my front doorknob, a gift from my friend Linda who is a jewelry artist. I read her message on my phone:

> *Wear it when you go to chemo. Look at each bead; they're all different. Put a happy thought with each one or someone you love. It's to keep your mind on happy things, places, and people.*
>
> **Me:** *I'll wear it like a rosary of love.*

Happy thoughts can lift my spirits but not my body off this couch. The hardest part of living with cancer so far is chemo's impact on my energy level—if there was a cuff to measure mine, it would register zippo. A breast cancer survivor reassures me with these words:

> *I was a couch potato during chemo.*

That will never be me, I thought at first. Now I understand what she meant. I'm supposed to keep moving, but I don't feel like it. A positive attitude will carry me far but not too far from the sofa. The oncology nurse who administered my first dose of chemo warned me of the sudden onset of fatigue: "Be prepared to need more rest."

Stillness feels foreign, like I'm in a place where I can't read the street signs. Taking it easy is like fumbling with a new language— awkward and unnatural. Psalm 46:10 tells me to cease striving, to be still, to place my restlessness in God's hands. The trouble is, rest is about *being* instead of *doing*, and I'm a doer. Simply *being* is boring and frustrating but nevertheless nonnegotiable during this season. Chemotherapy shifts all my gears into low.

But thinking of rest as gift—not something I'm forced to do— changes everything. I may try to ignore the commandment to rest, but it's built into the universe and I can't survive without it. My son Brett recently posted a request for prayers for peace and healing for me on Facebook. I imagine the kindness, good thoughts, and prayers sent my way are still rippling, vibrating through space and out into eternity, then circling back like a boomerang. I close my eyes and find rest easier in this wide ocean of goodwill.

> **Me:** *Journaled, slept, watched* Downton Abbey *season one, first episode. First chemo down, fifteen to go ... lots of time for more episodes.*
>
> **High school friend:** *Watch it while you rest and heal!*
>
> **Friend:** *Rest. In. God.*
>
> **Me:** *And I'm learning—Rest. Like. God.*
>
> **Julie:** *The first treatment is behind you. Please allow yourself to rest, Mama.*

Remember Jesus, serenely sleeping in a rocking fishing boat on the Sea of Galilee while the quaking disciples panicked? A fierce wind from the Mediterranean cut through a narrow mountain pass beyond the lake, and those terrified fishermen shook Jesus awake. Unrattled, he addressed the elements: "Peace! Be still" (Mark 4:39). Storms threatened and waves crashed, but Jesus spoke peace into the storm. I want to rest in the deep peace of Jesus and pass it on to others. Lord God, please bring restorative rest to my body, mind, and spirit. Your invitation for us to come to you is never outdated.

I whisper breath prayers of rest and peace, fingering each bead on my rosary bracelet in a ritual of trust.

All will be well.

THE COLOR PINK

"They are no longer two, but one flesh."

—MARK 10:8, NIV

Jim appeared at the top of the steps grinning, his damp, long-sleeve white shirt and blue jeans stained raspberry pink. It was eighty-six degrees.

Jim has filled many roles over the last five decades, but this is a new one: chief berry picker. With a dishpan half full of plump, perfect raspberries to prove it, he's become my berry hero. Picking berries is supposed to be my job, my joy. Jim's dad planted twelve raspberry canes on the lowest part of our lot more than thirty years ago. I've been the master of the berry patch ever since. The canes multiplied into the hundreds—two hedges bearing bright red goodness, summer and autumn, until the first hard freeze. Sometimes I'm still picking at Thanksgiving, like Mom and I did the autumn Dad died.

Berry picking is a way to breathe in God's goodness. I have nothing to focus on but the next berry, the perfect setting for contemplating the Spirit within. Small as they are, berries are part of God's overall plan: "The land produced vegetation: plants bearing seed according to their kinds and trees bearing fruit with seed in it according to their kinds. And God saw that it was good" (Gen. 1:12, NIV). Yes, Lord, very good.

One overcast morning while Brett was visiting, we hiked down to the raspberry patch. I was covered head to foot to avoid the sun, which is toxic for folks on chemo. Mistake. I felt nause-ated from the heat by the time I made it back up to the house, leaving the guys to work on their own.

When I posted on Facebook that berries were ripe, friends came picking. A local college student responded and brought her parents and grandmother visiting from Shanghai. They carried baskets and seemed to have a good time traipsing to our berry hedge, surrounded by summer greenery. The student posted:

> *We went to Jan's place to pick raspberries!*
> *After she told me raspberry is good for fighting*
> *against breast cancer, I just want to pick fresh*
> *raspberries every day for her.*

God provided people from the far side of the world to join their story to ours for an afternoon. Similarly, the way Jim has stepped up blesses my heart daily. Believe me, berries are just the beginning. I won't mention the litter box. He's my hands, my feet, my back.

One morning Jim was pushing firewood through the wood splitter, mulling over my diagnosis, grinding the words *breast can-cer* through his heart and soul. He ended up with a mountain of wood and then went inside to record his thoughts. Later he shared "The Color Pink" with me:

> To me, pink was a neutral color. Sure, sports teams donned pink socks, shoes, gloves, hats, or whatever—fans even waved pink terrible towels— all to promote awareness and support the fight against breast cancer. The fight, however, really wasn't my fight, and I figured those "pink" mer-chandisers were making a killing (perhaps a poor

choice of words). Pink was a nondescript color until my wife, the love of my life, my best friend, the mother of my three children, was diagnosed with breast cancer.

Before now, colon cancer had most of my attention. My father and his father before him succumbed to that wretched disease. I've been proactive with diet and screenings, alert to the possibility it might be a fight in the future. At this moment though, breast cancer is Public Enemy Number One. From the time my wife found that lump, it seems we've boarded a train. I say "we" because we have boarded this train together, and it has taken us on a ride we hadn't scheduled—through mammograms, sonograms, biopsies, and a whole village of medical professionals. Sometimes it feels like a bullet train but then, especially as we waited for pathology and prognosis, something much, much slower.

I hate seeing Jan have to go through this, and I don't relish the battle ahead. We are people of faith and know we are not on our own. Family, friends, and the peace of God surround us. The fight is on! Pink is no longer without meaning. It just got personal.

Thanks, Honey, for traveling with me on this unexpected journey.

All will be well.

WHERE DOES IT HURT?

We know love by this, that he laid down his
life for us—and we ought to lay down our lives
for one another. How does God's love abide in
anyone who has the world's goods and sees a
brother or sister in need and yet refuses help?

—1 JOHN 3:16-17

When I tumbled off my bike as a kid somebody always asked, "Where does it hurt?" One fall stands out.

Looking oh-so-cool, I zoomed down Hillcrest Avenue with hands in my pockets, free as the breeze. Too late I realized I should have started braking halfway down. A pile of rocks awaited me at the end of the street where a house was under construction. In a split-second decision, I rolled left, knowing I'd land on the new macadam road, which was hard but still better than loose rocks. No damage done—except to my pride, elbow, and knees.

"Where does it hurt?" Mother asked, seeing me drag my bike into the garage. Healing began with her question because of the loving care in her voice.

After my first dose of chemo I landed in the hospital for three days with a bowel obstruction, combined with a nonexistent white cell count. Each nurse and doctor asked the same question: "Where does it hurt?" Their caring contributed to my healing.

As a parent, I asked my kids the same question—sometimes daily, depending on the rate of bumps and bruises. Our trio of children learned to ride in front of our house, beginning with a Big Wheel and graduating to a bike with training wheels. It took Mom, Dad, or an older sibling running alongside to coax the newbie on. Eventually, with a final push from behind, one more independent rider wobbled down the road, eyes wide in pride and wonder. The hardest part for me was knowing, as sure as apples drop from the tree, that at some point they would stumble and smack the ground. Then came the question: "Where does it hurt?"

The other hard thing was knowing the day would come when they'd ride off on their own, down the hill and out of sight. They, like me, hankered for bigger adventures. Now they live far beyond that hilltop road.

Big Sis gave Jim and me a globe before our son was born. It seemed like a weird baby gift back then, but now I hope that dusty sphere was spun enough times to teach our kids that a universe lies beyond our circle of hills. While instructing our children how to pedal or swim, I often worried if they would learn the important things. Was I teaching them to care for others? One thing's for sure—as they grew and their worlds expanded, they taught me about accepting those who don't fit into a box neatly labeled "People Like Me."

I wish I could ask our world, "Where does it hurt?" and somehow say everything will be all right. But that's already been done for us. The Beloved is near, even as we crash due to our own delusions. Jesus takes on our hurts, makes them his own, and carries them to the throne room of heaven. Mourning over Jerusalem and its navel-gazing leaders, this young Jewish rabbi shook his head and said, "How often I wanted to gather your children together, the way a hen gathers her chicks under her wings, and you were unwilling" (Matt. 23:37, NASB).

Where does it hurt?

Everywhere.

If we hope for change anywhere, it begins with caring about those who are different from us—caring more than fearing what separates us. Like Jesus did. Caring because others are no less human, hurting, or deserving than we are.

A reader sends this message:

> I took my friend to her chemotherapy
> treatments, and thank God she is fine now after
> two bouts of breast cancer. No matter what
> your circumstances, you can still be kind. I live
> by this.

It's something I can—and must—do daily. Chemo or not. I stroll the road with my Palestinian neighbor, sharing stories and concerns like women have done throughout time. Her smiling son cycles beside us as we take small steps together on the same street where my children learned to ride. If they were still kids, this young fellow would be their playmate.

All will be well.

BECOMING REAL

"The LORD does not look at the things
people look at. People look at the outward
appearance, but the LORD looks at the heart."

—1 SAMUEL 16:7, NIV

Doctors say hair loss is the hardest thing for cancer patients. I remember that, exchanging smiles with women wearing wigs and hats, waiting for chemotherapy, wondering how they cope and who they were before this disease changed their lives forever.

My hospital's women's center provides a haven to sit at a vanity and try on wigs, hats, and more. All free. After experimenting with a pile, I choose a perky little highlighted wig. It's itchy and therefore occupies a stand on my dresser, except when I leave the house. Always one of the tallest girls, I've worn flamboyant hats since I was little. Now I hope they add a little spice, a distraction from my missing locks.

On days when not much helps, I can opt for make-believe, pretending to be well and happy, handling hair loss and everything else with nonchalance. Pretending isn't always bad. As a first grader, I pretended to read *Dick and Jane* until one afternoon in the school library the words came alive on the page, and I read for the very first time. Sometimes pretending carries me along until what's real can heal. Today I played dress-up at the bathroom mirror, drawing lines for my missing eyebrows, trying on new turquoise earrings, stuffing my bra with a cotton sock.

Later, when Jim saw me reading in the recliner, he tilted his head in approval and smooched my bald head.

Going public with breast cancer opens doors to connect with others going through challenging times, but it's one of the hardest things I've ever done. And it comes with risks. Some friends on similar journeys are quieter, avoiding the label, "that woman with cancer."

Is that how people see me? Does it matter if they do?

> **Friend:** *Thank you for being so transparent. To God be the glory!*

Fiona, one of the teenagers from a Kenyan family we consider our own, reminded me that we're more than the sum of our ailments, accomplishments, or looks, when she asked, "Why does it matter what people think of you, Grandma?"

A good question. I didn't have a good answer. I didn't tell Fiona about a lifetime of feeling like I've messed up, of struggling to measure up. Until now, I didn't realize cancer would push my self-esteem issues to the surface. What I know is that, like the well-worn *Velveteen Rabbit* we read about as children, I want to be real—with hair or without. The Skin Horse explained what real means:

> "Generally, by the time you are Real, most of your hair has been loved off, and your eyes drop out, and you get loose in the joints and very shabby. But these things don't matter at all, because once you are Real you can't be ugly, except to people who don't understand."[4]

We spend a lot of time and effort inventing false selves we desperately hope others will like; then perhaps we'll like ourselves better too. That's the honest answer to Fiona's question. But cancer is helping me detach from my false self—a self that takes too much energy. The good news is that Jim isn't the only one giving me smooches. My family and friends love me as I am, maybe even more than before.

All will be well.

The Practice of Detachment

"Where your treasure is,
there your heart will be also."

—MATTHEW 6:21, NIV

Detachment is an unfamiliar faith discipline to many, yet Jesus detached every time he turned away from the allure of the world. I practice it by focusing on God's goodness. Detachment teaches me I need less stuff, whether it's family treasures, ingrained attitudes, or constant busyness. I detach from things, worries, and opinions by visualizing myself taking a step to the side and mentally releasing whatever I'm clutching, whatever distracts me. Then I see myself floating unburdened down a sparkling stream, drifting lightly in a current of peace.

Some of the first Christians to practice detachment as a discipline may have been those who moved to the desert to live monastic lives. The Bible implores us to set our minds on things above, not on earth. This means deliberately choosing what to think about, even while doing humdrum chores like the dishes or laundry. This practice invites us to visually place thoughts and feelings in God's hands, trusting the mind of Christ to guide our own.

Detaching creates space to attach myself to Jesus. I detach throughout the day—when anxiety threatens to tangle my nerves, while blood is drawn, when I'm forced to skip a gathering because little kids will be racing around, carrying germs that could attack my lowered immune system. Early on, as a breast cancer survivor,

I relinquished a small, warm breast and my thick, wavy hair, knowing I'm not defined by either them or by cancer.

Sometimes I find myself looking around my home and asking myself, *What can I get rid of?* Parting reluctantly with books, clothes, dishes, and memorabilia demonstrates how emotionally attached I am to things that connect me to other people, especially those who have died. I've learned that saying goodbye to things doesn't mean I forget those who gave them to me. I'm now able to send precious items off with a blessing: "Bring joy to someone else!" Now, when someone admires something, I'm apt to say, "Here, please give it a good home."

Practicing detachment is about more than giving away our possessions. It's also about

- Releasing emotional ties to things, thoughts, and activities.
- Surrendering hopes and fears to God.
- Recognizing we don't need to hold an opinion about everything.
- Accepting that we don't have to be right or perfect to be content.
- Forbidding cancer or _____ (fill in the blank) from dominating our thinking.

One evening when I was exhausted, I distinctly heard the Spirit caution me, "Don't try to do too much." It was a sacred call to detach from commitments that didn't seem right for me at that point in my journey. Paradoxically, when I pause to listen to what God *is* calling me to do and be, windows open that were previously shut

Is God calling you to explore the discipline of detachment?

* * *

Surely all of us have something we ought to let go of, whether it's a coat that no longer fits or an attitude that drags us down. In addition to passing along items you no longer need to people who could use them, consider which habits or tendencies you might need to let go of as well. Talk to God about what you need to surrender from a personal perspective. What no longer serves you? Picture yourself placing whatever dominates your thinking or clutters your life right now into the hands of Jesus. Trust that it's no longer your responsibility. It might be hard at first to surrender those attachments that have been part of your life for so long. The more you return, again and again, to detachment, the easier it will become. Invite God to help you concentrate on what really matters so that you might feel freer, all the while creating more space for family, friends, and faith.

BRIDGES AND INTERLUDES

Let everything that has breath praise the LORD.

—PSALM 150:6, NIV

When I was a kid, I'd lie awake giddy the night before school let out for the summer. What joy to fly through those big glass doors with three long months stretching before me, custom-made for biking, swimming, and devouring books in my shady backyard. Of course, school days always returned in September—summer was only an interlude. A passing season for building sandcastles and memories.

I was asked to speak at a cancer fundraiser and wanted to include a comment about bridges. Out of curiosity, I asked Tina, my church's organist who also happens to be a breast cancer survivor, the difference between an interlude and a bridge in music. "An interlude can be a longer piece of music and stand on its own. In a play, an interlude may be used while the scenery is changed," she said. "A bridge connects two pieces of the same piece."

Cancer has changed the scenery for me. Taking me into sterile settings for treatments. Forcing me out of the sun I crave, limiting much of my time outdoors to a covered breezeway because sunlight doesn't mix well with chemotherapy. I'm too early in the game yet to know if cancer will be merely an interlude or become a bridge. In music, a bridge comes in the middle of a piece, connecting two sections of music. When you hear a bridge it always means something's coming up next, so I'm hoping cancer is a bridge to something better.

Jim led contemporary worship at our church for fourteen years, filling our home with praise as he practiced music week after week, year after year. He said a bridge adds interest to a song, especially when there are multiple verses: "A bridge takes you somewhere; an instrumental interlude provides a pause." Right now, I'm in pause mode, but I sure as heck don't plan to stay here.

During the worship segment of a praise gathering Jim and I attended, we sang a song based on Psalm 18:2: "The LORD is my rock, my fortress, and my deliverer, my God, my rock in whom I take refuge, my shield, and the horn of my salvation, my stronghold." Afterward, I told Jim it's time to fill our home with praise music again.

An old hymn that energizes me is Martin Luther's "A Mighty Fortress Is Our God." It is based on the scripture, "God is our refuge and strength, A very ready help in trouble" (Ps. 46:1, NASB). We're meant to sing from our souls and shout from our hearts that God is our high tower, a stronghold where we're sheltered and unafraid. When we repeatedly sing the Word, we imprint it indelibly on our hearts.

I discovered that our brains are vast music storehouses when I worked with patients with dementia. Residents who could barely talk still loved to sing around tables and gather in wheelchairs for church. The song they requested more than any other was "Jesus Loves Me." It stirred me to see folks nearing life's end sit up a little straighter and lift their chins to sing those lyrics.

On days I lacked the stamina to unload both racks of the dishwasher at one time, I found refuge in music. Sometimes I spread my arms wide and swirled by the big, glass sliding doors in our living room, making my dance a prayer. As I moved, I remembered running out those old school doors, swinging wide into summer vacation. Psalm 150 says praising God with music and dance is a prescription for healthier days, and I felt better when I did. Thankfully no one could see me but crows and sparrows flying by, and if they were laughing, I'll never know.

All will be well.

SISTER STRENGTH

Praise be to the God and Father of our Lord Jesus
Christ, the Father of compassion and the God of
all comfort, who comforts us in all our troubles,
so that we can comfort those in any trouble with
the comfort we ourselves receive from God.

—2 CORINTHIANS 1:3-4, NIV

Me: *My hair's falling out.*

Big Sis: *One day at a time. If it prevents
another breakout of cancer, it's worth it. You
are loved!*

Breast cancer survivor: *I found it a great
excuse to get big earrings.*

Sounds reasonable—retail therapy has to be more fun than
chemotherapy.

Me to daughter: *Going out to buy big hoops.*

Daughter: *Hoops?*

Me, later: *Earrings. I bought five pairs.*

* * *

I sat on a stool on our deck. Jim, my Mr. Fix-It, who can repair most anything by watching a YouTube video, buzzed a razor around my scalp. His eyes filled—perhaps because cancer is one thing not even love can fix. An oncologist had forewarned me, "You'll cry one more time, when you lose your hair." I did. Silently, like Jim.

Compassion, like love, is unlimited. Marilyn and I write our way through our feelings. We live three states apart but tune in to each other like some people tune in to a radio station. I didn't grasp how deeply she felt my losses until she sent me a piece she'd written to help her process the situation:

> Four little words, *I'm losing my hair*, hit like a double-barreled shotgun, hurting me twice as deeply than if they'd been my own. Janet and I sometimes squabbled while growing up. I owned the privilege of fighting with—and on occasion for—my identical twin. When she hurt, I hurt. If she succeeded, I felt pride. Decades ago, we hit our stride as grown up sister-friends. Birth gave us a shared history, and faith offers a shared future. In between, constant "twin-cidences" bound us together. We both married guys named Jim, twice gave birth days apart.
>
> Our biggest difference was our health. I was the one struggling, carrying a backpack of pain into our sixties, when Janet called from her kayak in the middle of a lake one morning.
>
> "Can't imagine what it's like to live without pain," I said wistfully.

"I can't imagine what it's like to live with it," she answered, so softly I could almost hear her paddling through the water.

Now I try to imagine what it's like to be more concerned about saving my life than my hair. I naively thought breast cancer would never strike my sisters or me. Janet, especially, seemed too strong to be touched by it. It felt as though I began holding my breath when she told me of her diagnosis, and I only released it after she first wrote the words, "All will be well." It reminded me of a time when my young daughter plunged down steep steps. I held my breath in that moment too, only exhaling when her Uncle Jim Woodard caught her in his strong arms. All was well.

Confronting cancer's grief and fear, I'm strengthened by Janet's faith, trusting our heavenly Father to offer us both the refuge of his love. "The eternal God is a hiding place, And underneath are the everlasting arms" (Deut. 33:27, NASB).

***

I have sisters by birth, marriage, and choice. Compassionate women who walk with me—in person or in my heart—and help me bear the heavy load of cancer.

All will be well.

GOOD MEDICINE

Like the oil of gladness,
friendship is sweet to the soul.

—PROVERBS 27:9, ap

Me: *Going home for my fiftieth high school
reunion.*

Friend: *We'll be praying for you!*

Me: *Thanks! Just got my white blood count—it's
perfect!*

A decent white-blood cell count meant I could spend the weekend around old buddies in my hometown, less wary of catching germs that could land me back in the hospital. I was resting in my hotel bed before our class cookout, glad to have my itchy wig off for a few minutes, when Marilyn unexpectedly opened the door. Her eyes welled with tears.

"Oh," she said.

"It's okay," I responded. She was the only one to see me bareheaded that weekend. Most classmates never suspected my perky little wig wasn't the real thing. I laughed out loud when one guy said I hadn't changed since high school.

"What's your secret?"

"I'm a plastic surgeon," Jim joked, not missing a beat.

The night of the banquet, I left the hall for a break and found a couple glancing through photographs, uncertain if they'd stay to eat or slip away unnoticed because they hadn't registered for the event. It took Carol, another classmate, saying, "Of course you're staying and sitting at our table!" to convince them they belonged. I wish I'd done that. She turned faith into action, demonstrating what women have always done, instinctively nurturing others.

A short time later that's how I felt—nurtured—when I spotted my best high school friend across the crowd. What followed was the longest, fiercest hug of my life.

"I didn't know if you'd come," Leticia said, pausing. "After I heard about your cancer." With a broad smile, Leticia, an exchange student from Brazil, had quickly won our hearts all those years ago at school. We sat beside each other in American government class; evenings might find us at a kitchen table, books open. There were sleepovers, football games, youth retreats, and teenage talks about how we somehow fit into God's universe. Leticia stretched my worldview. Because of her, I taught American history before my babies came along and for decades have welcomed a host of international students through my front door. Transformed by her time in America, she was inspired to teach English in Rio.

Following our reunion, I needed extra rest but was refreshed by contact with old friends. Years and distance mean little when it comes to the power of friendship. Although the reunion was the only time we've spoken in the last fifty years, Joy, a nurse who sang at my wedding, has sent me a card and prayers every month since she learned of my diagnosis.

Friends are good medicine, and they remind me that joy spreads every time I reach out with love. Show me how to do that today, Lord.

All will be well.

TEND AND BEFRIEND

See what great love the Father has lavished on
us, that we should be called children of God!

—1 JOHN 3:1, NIV

My eyes brimmed when I opened the package. Inside was a
flowered cotton headscarf, a gift from Jennifer, my dear friend
Sandy's daughter, and a note. Their family had moved to Texas
thirty years earlier, and I hadn't seen Jennifer since. I was surprised she remembered me until I read this: "Mom was a warrior. I think she would like you to have it. Please wear it and think
of her. She is standing in your corner, cheering you on. May her
memory and spirit strengthen your determination to win this
fight for your life."

Wearing it now, I catch my reflection on my laptop screen
and recall Sandy's face, her eyes holding mine when she removed
her wig in my living room on her last visit to Pennsylvania. She
trusted the strength of our friendship to help her through that
very private reveal. I knelt beside her chair and hugged her.
We've loved each other across time, space, and now eternity. We
couldn't know then that someday I would go bald from chemotherapy too. After I wrote about the power of friendship, another
woman battling for her health posted this:

> *Wouldn't be here today without my friends!*
> *They carried me, physically and spiritually,*
> *when I couldn't!*

In the midst of cancer, I have this feeling we're all created to make life better in some way for others. I'm grateful to be a writer who can search for signs of hope and pass them along. It gives me a reason to get up in the morning. A reader posted this:

Our Lord's love resonates through your words
and sings of his love for each of us!

* * *

When I returned to school at fifty-eight, I learned about how women support one another in simple and powerful ways. In one of my classes I was introduced to the work of Dr. Shelley Taylor and a team of researchers who described the "tend and befriend" stress response in females.[5] At last, there was a sensible model for stressed-out women like me. Tend and befriend applies to those of us not fast enough to outrun our adversaries, nor strong enough to fight them off. Instinctively, we females tend to circle our wagons, instead of taking a heart-thumping "fight or flight" approach. When threatened, women are likely to band together. (In my case, it's usually over a cup of tea.) Or we stick around and tend to the most vulnerable who can't run either—the youngest, oldest, and most frail among us.

Cancer is my great adversary, my greatest stressor by a mile. Other women have encircled me with their care in scores of ways (sharing gallons of tea, for example). I know firsthand how friends lift my spirits so that I can make it through the day.

* * *

Jesus was devoted to his friends too. The love he shared with a young fellow named John shows how friendship changes people.

John was all bluster and thunder when Jesus first met him. He tried to reserve the best seat in heaven and wanted to call down fire to destroy a village of folks when he didn't like their behavior. I wish I could have seen the look on Jesus' face when John said that. Spending three years with Jesus transformed John into an intimate friend whose words on love transform us today. With time, he learned to listen for God's voice.

In his first letter, John penned, "We love because he first loved us" (1 John 4:19, NIV). At the Last Supper, John laid his head upon Jesus' breast and could almost hear the heartbeat of God; how that tender moment must have comforted both of them.

Anyone in pain or who suffers knows how isolating those feelings can be. At times I need space and want to be alone, yet I am designed to reflect God's image, whose eternal essence as the Three in One is relational. Jesus turned things upside down when he became human, wanting more than anything for us to know his father like he did. That's the heart behind the Incarnation. John 1:14 describes it like this: "The Word became a human being and lived here with us. We saw his true glory, the glory of the only Son of the Father. From him all the kindness and all the truth of God have come down to us" (CEV).

When we love Jesus like John did, we enter into the eternal flow of the Trinity. God's goodness is fleshed out in the here and now through the hands, feet, and hearts of family, neighbors, friends, doctors, nurses, and even strangers. There is little to compare to knowing others will be there for us no matter what.

Love, like my bandanna from an old friend, covers a multitude of losses.

All will be well.

RETREAT

A bright red spot in a backyard tree caught my eye. A cardinal? No. A sassafras leaf. Fall is coming.

In spring I feared what summer might bring. As late August brushes sky and field in amber gold, a fresh mindset is unfolding, like a butterfly emerging from a chrysalis. Not that I've seen many butterflies this summer, as I've been mostly indoors, looking from the inside out. I've yet to spot a monarch, but one day when I had the energy to walk the dog with Jim, he introduced me to their tiny solitary white eggs on the underside of milkweed leaves. They're so small that he uses a miniature handheld microscope to view their delicate pattern. Monarchs, like hope, have seemingly impossible beginnings yet evolve into something that inspires me to look up.

Small encounters with the natural world are a metaphor for the butterfly effect, the fanciful idea that minuscule influences— like a butterfly beating its wings—have an impact on climatic conditions a world away. Whether or not this happens, nature's small gifts have enriched this summer of my retreat. One of them, blue chicory, edges our road like little welcome signs. Another, a goldfinch, perches on a pink coneflower wavering in the cool breeze. Its fleeting yellow presence tells me purple bull thistles must have gone to seed, transforming them into goldfinch feeders. Sure enough, there's a prickly thistle bowed over, heavy with the burden of its abundance. It causes me to bow as well before the Creator of these common splendors.

I took a class in my spiritual formation program in which we studied the lives of desert fathers and mothers, called *abbas* and *ammas*, taught by Roberta Bondi, professor emerita at Emory's Candler School of Theology. These people chose life in the desert over the opulence of newly Christianized Rome. They weren't seeking more stuff and bigger adventures. These don't settle my heart either. Retreating with Jesus redirects me to what is life-giving, like Jim's tiny microscope urging me to refocus my eyes.

The idea of retreating takes me to the woods, remembering my kids splashing in streams and singing around a campfire, swatting away mosquitoes. I think of other "re" words like *renew, restore, replenish, repent*. Some pull my thoughts toward home. Retreating at its best—even with mosquitoes—requires slowing down, quieting the pace of my noisy busyness. I need retreats not only because chemo treatments make my mind foggy but also because I have a hurried heart.

The word *hurry* brings *dash* to mind. *Haste. Push. Rush.* My heart jumps at the thought; I've spent a lot of time careening through life over the years. The opposite? *Calm. Quiet. Rest. Hush.* Hard for this Type-A, yackety-yak woman. But interior retreats take me from the first list of words to the second. It's like kayaking on a raging creek that branches off into smooth waters.

Stillness and silence open doors for meditation. My breezeway provides a perfect sanctuary for me to meditate on warm afternoons, with music provided by Carolina wrens perched in the branches of a towering blue spruce. For decades, that tree protected the breezeway from rain and snow. Now I feel sheltered by faith and prayers from the emotional blasts of living with cancer.

> **Me:** My energy's at zero right now, so I'm
> learning to do nothing and to do it well!
>
> **Linda, an old Bible study friend:** We humans
> think we have to be busy all the time. God
> is pleased when we can just "be." Enjoy the
> "being" process.

Focusing on a single red leaf helps me do that. And I'm still on the lookout for a monarch.

All will be well.

The Practice of Meditation

"Be still, and know that I am God!"

—PSALM 46:10

Meditation is at the heart of most faith disciplines. It is a doorway into God's presence. Why do it? Because the Word commands it (see Joshua 1:8); it deepens our experience of community with one another and the Trinity (see 2 Corinthians 13:11-14); it enriches our souls (see Proverbs 4:20-22); and it helps us love others (see Mark 12:28-31). When I think of meditation, I think of Jesus—of his time alone with his Father in the desert for forty days, of his habit of going off to pray on private retreats. If I want to be like Jesus, I need to follow his sandals to lonely places. I imagine Jesus hungered for those singular times with God. Being together fed his soul sweet fruit that nourished and equipped him for ministry and sacrifice as nothing else could.

The simplest definition of *meditation* is listening to God. It takes stillness, solitude, and silence, turning off the incessant chatter of our culture and intentionally spending time with the Sacred Three. Even children need healthy solitude in safe settings, alone with their thoughts and a growing wonder about the world and God.

Setting aside a stretch of time for silent meditation doesn't work for everybody. I think of caregivers and of busy parents, scrambling to compress care for kids, work, and home into twenty-four-hour days. As the parent of three kids with a husband who traveled for his work, I went through seasons when I shot off arrow prayers between the mayhem with little energy or time to enter into the Holy of Holies. Of course, God understands and is no less present in our chaos than in our calm.

I've meditated upon Andrei Rublev's fifteenth-century icon "The Trinity," which portrays the scene in Genesis when Abraham and Sarah (both out of sight) offered hospitality to mysterious visitors. The title suggests the guests are Father, Son, and Spirit. Study this Russian icon and with a little imagination you'll see there is an empty seat at the table. That seat is reserved for you. The Sacred Three welcome us to the table, into the family, and into the family conversation. My friends and family know I struggle to overcome the habit of interrupting others; being in the presence of these gracious listeners as I meditate upon this icon makes me yearn to be more like them. One way to do that is by setting my mind upon the Word and storing it in my heart. (See "The Practice of Praying God's Word.")

Breathing fresh air helps me meditate too. Jesus spent most of his days outdoors, witnessing God's paintbrush on the green hills of Galilee, in the chilly winds sweeping across the sea, and in the rose-colored skies over desolate Judean mountains. He probably slept on the ground, contemplating the stars, recalling with a smile how God scattered them, like diamonds, in space. I hope I can ponder God's goodness in the crisp air of creation until the end of my days.

* * *

Through the ancient art of meditation, we come to know not only God better but also ourselves. Start by incorporating just five or ten minutes of silence into your daily routine. Find a comfortable spot to sit, preferably with your back straight and your feet on the floor so you feel stable and grounded. Don't have an agenda beyond settling yourself and listening for God. As you become accustomed to the silence, you can increase the time of your meditation as appropriate for your temperament and your lifestyle. Quieting our hearts, minds, and bodies takes practice. But all you have to do is show up. God is already there, waiting for you in the silence.

THE MONKEY
AND THE CAT

My dear friends, stand firm and don't be shaken.
Always keep busy working for the Lord. You know
that everything you do for him is worthwhile.

—1 CORINTHIANS 15:58, CEV

I would have missed two weathered carvings inside Iona Abbey on my Celtic pilgrimage if my roommate, Judy, had not pointed them out. High above the Communion table, inside a window wall as I remember, are rough images of a monkey and a cat.

For hundreds of years, Iona, an isle off the Scottish coast, was the site of a Benedictine monastery. In the twentieth century, the abbey was rebuilt after gradually falling into ruin following the Reformation. Why the carvings? They represent two sides of Benedictine life—and ours as people of faith: activity (the monkey) and stillness (the cat).

Most of my life there has been a feline underfoot. It just feels right to have a kitty rubbing my legs or draped over my shoulders in a chair, silken as my grandmother's fox furs (a somewhat silly and now objectionable fashion statement from an earlier era). Cancer's heavy cloud hung over me when I began journaling about it in the local newspaper; often, I extended my arms and hands over our kitty, Pia, curled on my lap, to reach my keyboard. Her intuition told her I needed extra comfort. I didn't know it, but she did.

In the mornings, Pia's rough pink tongue would awaken me, licking my face, announcing it was time for breakfast. I envied her ability to stretch every vertebra in her back in slow motion. Her presence calmed my restlessness and slowed my heart rate when I held her close. Then the vet found cancer in her jaw. After sixteen years, it was hard to say goodbye.

When Iona Abbey was originally built, perhaps after watching a tabby delicately bathe herself, some monk was inspired to carve a cat to portray the tranquil side of his life's calling. It is in contemplation that we grow in wisdom, worship, and prayer, making it easier to release our fists when they're squeezed with worries.

Then there's that spunky monkey, high against another wall, begging for our attention. If only he could talk! We'll never know if the same artist chiseled his image into rock. This fellow represents all the activities vital to surviving on a tiny isle, surrounded by crashing waves. Those isolated there farmed, tended sheep, spun wool, repaired fishing nets, and performed a thousand other chores. Unlike those monks and nuns, I'm at a point where I pretty much do what I want (no one forces busyness upon me, except myself). When I cram too much into a day or week, life becomes like my book collection that is stacked everywhere. Too much activity, like too many books, is overwhelming and signals I'm overloaded.

Late one night, Jim and I returned from a visit to the old rustic cabin we inherited in the Finger Lakes region of upstate New York. Despite my cancer, we had worked diligently cleaning and organizing. The next night, I dreamed we were up to our knees in some sort of project outside the cabin when we heard God calling. It was a Genesis 3:8 moment (when God walked in the Garden, calling to Adam and Eve). You'd think this voice would cause us to at least look up. Instead, one of us (was it me?) said, "Not now," and we continued on our task. Awake, I can't imagine the audacity of telling the Almighty not now—yet how often does my lifestyle do just that, ignoring God's voice for my own priorities?

A few days after Jim and I returned from the cabin, my yoga instructor said to quiet our "monkey minds" and focus on being present exactly where we were. I smiled at the image—my thoughts often wander as persistently as monkeys swinging from branch to branch, forcing me time and again to lasso them back into the present.

I'm glad my roommate pointed out those carvings to me. Now I mull over them as a cancer warrior, seeing them as signposts, guiding my way. Lord of work and prayer, of service and contemplation, thank you that centuries ago some wise person etched small creatures into stone that still teach us today.

All will be well.

WRESTLING MATCH

Why am I discouraged?
Why am I restless?
I trust you!
And I will praise you again
because you help me,
and you are my God.

—PSALM 42:11, CEV

In the early hours, before my eyes fully open, it takes a minute to remember.

Breast cancer.

My eyes shut again, as if that will change reality.

At the county fair, I weave my way through a parade of life-size panels featuring sixty-seven Pennsylvania women fighting breast cancer, one for each county in the state. I go early while it's still cool and quiet, hoping to come home empowered by their stories. Instead, seeing their efforts and brave smiles drains me; I leave after reading only a few. Cancer has yet to pin me down, but some days it's hard to watch others in the ring.

* * *

The Bible is full of people who struggled with family issues, people issues, God issues. People like Jacob, who grappled with a mysterious Presence through an endless night. Shirt soaking, hip

aching, Jacob demanded a blessing before releasing his oppo-
nent. The Lord, who knew his heart, honored his request. Jacob
became Israel that day, a wrestler who strove with God. (See
Genesis 32.) My faith is built upon generations who followed
Jacob and came to know this wilderness God through their suf-
ferings as much as in their blessings.

I may spend most of my days in a recliner right now but make
no mistake: I'm pressing fiercely into Jesus, feeling his muscle
tone, knowing him better in the heat of battle. Jim tells me that is
because it's impossible to wrestle from a distance.

> **Me, to cancer patient:** Real life is hard. My
> heart is with you!
>
> **Cancer patient, nearing the end:** Sometimes it
> is just really hard for us to see God's goodness
> in the moment.

Definitely. My grandson Eli watched *The Prince of Egypt*, the
story of Moses, while cuddling with his mama, down in New
Zealand. Later, Tara let me know Eli said, "Sometimes God
seems a little . . . demanding."

"Yes," replied Tara. "He does."

Jesus came to walk the road beside us and restore our relationship with God. The hard part of God—the part that we may
feel allows evil in the name of free will—is beyond us, or at least
beyond me. I seldom hear anything but one-size-fits-all explana-
tions for evil and pain, yet I have come to believe rejecting easy
answers in the face of suffering is as acceptable in Jesus' sight as
thanking him for his mysterious ways.

I was deliberating on this when Elizabeth dropped by for
breakfast. (She stopped to check on me, really.) She and I met

through a college program and have treated one another as family for years. She lost her parents when young, so she's called Jim and me Dad and Mum from the beginning. The six years she was separated from her family in Kenya due to war, poverty, and famine wove our stories into one. Being around her put things in perspective. The faith she inherited from her Maasai grandfather, a pioneer Christian, shines brighter than all the questions she wrestles with in the dark. Before leaving, she spoke a blessing upon us with each word in her lovely voice rising like sweet incense to God.

That was yesterday. In this morning's shadows, I wait for the sun to slip out of hiding, trusting God with a weary heart while my head mutters doubts. Jacob wrestled in the dark until a blessing came, then hobbled into the light. Like him, my limping faith keeps me going, enabling me to continue repeating my life mantra:

All will be well.

PRAYING PSALMS

Your word is a lamp to my feet
and a light to my path.

—PSALM 119:105

Four a.m. I throw back the sheet and reach for the foot of my scrolled metal bed frame. Feeling my way to the bathroom, I nod to an owl-shaped nightlight, who solemnly ignores me. We repeat this ritual, nightly. Thankful the dim glow doesn't switch on my brain's wake-up center, I pad back to bed, swallow my thyroid pill, and pray sleep returns.

"The LORD is my shepherd. . . . " drifts through my brain's wrinkled crevices.

A former pastor once said that if you read a psalm every day, then you'll know what God is like. On that advice, I'm reading and praying them through this round of chemotherapy. When I can get my chemo brain to focus, the Psalms shed light on God's character, guide my feet in the dark, and slow my tongue through the day.

In *A Shepherd Looks at Psalm 23*, author W. Phillip Keller tells of a shepherd deep in a cistern in Africa, furiously bailing water for thirsty sheep. I can see him, this shirtless, sweaty fellow, totally responsible for the animals in his charge. Then I read a line by Keller about *our* Good Shepherd that jumped off the page and splashed out of that African watering hole: "But it simply must be remembered that He is there with us in it."[6]

A needle in my chemo port sends potentially dangerous, potentially healing chemicals coursing through my veins. My Great Physician is in it with me.

"The LORD is my shepherd, I shall not want" (Ps. 23:1).

The oncologist said this chemo will be easier than the first. Not to argue, but I hear that many cancer patients acquire neuropathy, numbness and tingling in their hands and feet that can last forever. Fending this off, I hold frozen water bottles in gloved hands during hour-long injections—a home remedy if ever there was one. A nurse shakes her head as I murmur, "Eleven more times." My Companion is in it with me.

"He makes me lie down in green pastures" (Ps. 23:2).

Legs wrapped in heated blankets, feet bundled in heavy socks, I balance them on frozen milk cartons during these final chemo treatments. To avoid more thrush in my mouth, sore from earlier treatments, Jim spoons ice chips between my lips. I feel like a near-frozen little bird with its mouth open. My God is in it with me.

"He leads me beside still waters" (Ps. 23:2).

I hike a steep wooded path, far from anything remotely medical. The only needles are on the trees. Gratitude rises for blue skies, a shaggy white dog, and Jim, collector of red and brown mushrooms. My Creator is in it with me.

"He restores my soul. He leads me in right paths for his name's sake" (Ps. 23:3).

I wait to see a doctor, feet dangling, sure I have a urinary tract infection. My Healer is in it, with me.

"Even though I walk through the darkest valley, I fear no evil" (Ps. 23:4).

Cards arrive by the armful. So do bills. My Provider is in it with me.

"For you are with me; your rod and your staff—they comfort me" (Ps. 23:4).

I pray for my children, our fragmented country, and our fractured world. Trusting Jesus is in it with me. With us all.

"You prepare a table before me in the presence of my enemies; you anoint my head with oil; my cup overflows" (Ps. 23:5).

Whether my cup is full, cracked, or empty, my Shepherd is in it with me. I'm not alone.

"Surely goodness and mercy shall follow me all the days of my life, and I shall dwell in the house of the LORD my whole life long" (Ps. 23:6).

> **Sue, a breast cancer survivor and one of my students forty-five years ago:** Absolutely the exact words I needed to hear today.

Better, warmer days lie ahead.

All will be well.

The Practice of Praying God's Word

O come, let us worship and bow down,
let us kneel before the LORD, our Maker!

—PSALM 95:6

Like any faith discipline, our prayer life matures the more we remain in the presence of the Sacred Three. Prayer is more relational than merely listing petitions, as vital as that is. I'm forever grateful for the prayers lifted for me. If you wonder how to strengthen your conversation with God, praying the Word is a place to start. When we speak a psalm or other passage, we enter into God's thoughts, transforming our own.

Many praise songs are based on the Bible. When we tuck songs and verses in our hearts, they have a way of rising as prayers when we need them most. Jesus gave his followers the Lord's Prayer when they asked him to teach them to pray. Each time we pray it, we're praying scripture. Hundreds of verses express our desires and heartaches, especially the Psalms, which were originally written to be both prayed and sung.

An oncologist told me researchers have found positive ways to treat genes that have been altered by cancer. Even better, as we abide in the scriptures, I believe God's Word enhances our spiritual DNA. Try praying Psalm 91, making it yours by applying it to what is happening in your life today: "Whoever dwells in the shelter of the Most High will rest in the shadow of the Almighty.

I will say of the LORD, 'He is my refuge and my fortress, my God, in whom I trust'" (vv. 1-2, NIV).

A powerful New Testament passage to pray aloud is Philippians 2:1-11, a hymn of the early church that poignantly sings of the humility of Jesus and presents the essence of the gospel. At a time when harsh differences attempt to separate us, this prayer is a call to seek the mind and unity of Christ. "At the name of Jesus every knee should bend, in heaven and on earth and under the earth, and every tongue should confess that Jesus Christ is Lord, to the glory of God the Father" (Phil. 2:10-11). By praying aloud often enough, it will become second nature to return to those words as a mantra or a breath prayer.

* * *

Praying from the Bible lifts the Lord's words back to God in confidence that the entire Trinity listens and responds. The more you take such words to heart, the easier it will be for you to sense God's pledge to be ever present. Start with your favorite scripture, hymns, or other religious writings. Study them with your mind as well as your soul. Listen to what the words are telling you. Ask for help if you need assistance interpreting their meaning. Pray them aloud until they are committed to memory. Write them in your journal if that helps. Then move on to other parts of the Bible that maybe aren't as familiar to you. Praying God's Word can be both comforting and challenging. In the end, God is author of all.

GEMS IN THE CELLAR

We know that all things work together
for good for those who love God.

—ROMANS 8:28

A pressed oak leaf slipped out of a tree guidebook and into my hand. It sparked a memory of visiting a friend in the hospital one brilliant Sunday afternoon in September. Before going inside, I stepped into a stand of oaks and selected a shiny brown leaf. It wasn't much, but it was all I could offer as a last-minute gift. Lynn's bed was on the sixth floor and lacked a window view. She often said that brittle leaf was the only sign of fall she saw or touched that year.

A single leaf, remembered. Small things make a difference.

I believe everything crosses our paths for a reason, however close or far out in the universe the connection may be. One of those connections came to me as a little girl who suspected our soapstone cellar washtubs with flecks of mica secretly contained diamonds. (I read a lot of *Nancy Drew* mysteries back then.)

Stirring a pot on the stove one day long ago, Mother glanced at her hand and groaned, "My diamond is gone!" Detective that I was, I scampered downstairs and peered into a dark corner of a washtub. Sure enough, there was her precious diamond chip, waiting to be rescued before another laundry day washed it away. The girl who expected to find gems in the cellar still lives deep within me.

On a spiritual level, I believe God joins forces with us to shed light in dim corners. Friends say they're more grounded in faith with a clearer sense of selfhood because they've endured cancer, and so am I.

> **Linda, breast cancer survivor:** *I know it sounds strange, but I wouldn't trade this experience for anything.*
>
> **Woman with brain cancer:** *I'm making peace with cancer by focusing on what it is teaching me.*

It isn't easy to be positive when cancer marches around like a drill sergeant, intending to take charge. It's easier to surrender, starting with my sense of humor. But after talking on the phone with my nine-year-old grandson, Josiah, who lives on the other side of the world, I decided it was time to change my attitude.

"Grandma, I'll love you forever and ever!" he said. I want to ensure that there are many more talks and walks on this side of forever. In an act of holy resistance, I'm listing ten good things, ten life-giving truths, about cancer:

1. It strengthens ties with old friends and introduces me to new ones.
2. It surprises me through the kindness, love, and prayers of others.
3. It alerts me to hurting people and encourages me to extend a word or hand to them.
4. It helps me listen more deeply to others and myself.
5. It forces me to face fears I've ignored in the past.
6. It demands I give up on things I think define me.

7. It teaches me what is most important.
8. It shapes my faith into a sharp sword, cutting away what is frivolous and trivial.
9. It sets my heart and mind upon eternity.
10. It assures me again that nothing can separate me from God or from those I love.

These gems were mined from cancer's crucible, the last place I expected to find hidden riches. I began twelve new sessions of weekly chemotherapy last Tuesday. With new treatments come new risks as well as unforeseen grace to weather storms that blow my way. I welcome peace and thank God for sending it when I need it most.

All will be well.

MORE THAN A
MANNEQUIN

Carry each other's burdens, and in this
way you will fulfill the law of Christ.

—GALATIANS 6:2, NIV

I sit waiting for an empty dressing room at St. Vincent de Paul, my favorite thrift shop. My arms are laden with shirts, my energy zapped. *Maybe one of these will look right*, I tell myself. With a breast missing and no padding yet, it's hard to look or feel normal. Another bargain hunter glances in my direction, claps her hand over her mouth briefly, and then blurts out, "I thought you were a mannequin!"

We laugh together, but my shoulders cave. *I look like a mannequin?* Blame it on my wig and penciled eyebrows. I hug my pile of shirts and hope she doesn't notice a boob is missing.

***

It's been five months since my mastectomy. That procedure might have healed my body, but it did nothing to treat the flesh-and-blood fragility I feel. My heart seems closer to the surface now. It trembles like a ticking timepiece inside a hollow drum.

Electric-like impulses tingle across my chest. My numbed side, where fourteen lymph nodes were removed and nerves sliced, feels heavy, like a folded newspaper permanently tucked under my arm. Invariably, before sleep comes, my hand drifts to my rib cage where a small breast used to be. Size wasn't relevant to my risk of breast cancer. Countless strong women have come to terms with numbed bodies and frozen spirits after their flesh was cut away. I'm just beginning to defrost.

Others know this kind of loss. Jim once tried to describe his grief after having segments of two fingers amputated several decades ago. It wasn't the amount of tissue; it was feeling incomplete, fragmented. Something was missing. I didn't understand back then, but now I do. When he stood behind me at the bathroom mirror when I first glimpsed a deep purple gash on my chest, I turned away. His arms, wrapped around me, said more than words.

> **Joyce:** You are dressed in God's dignity and don't ever forget it, my sister survivor!

***

Grief's sharp knife can't sever me from this inner knowing that I'm part of something larger than myself. In 1624, English poet John Donne wrote, "No man is an island, Entire of itself. Every man is a piece of the continent, a part of the main. If a clod be washed away by the sea, Europe is the less."[7] His words trigger an image of relentless waves battering the sturdy Scottish coast and say that my broken bits of clay matter too.

> **A member of my Centering Prayer group, who has lost loved ones to cancer:** The most important principle of health is spiritual and emotional health. You have both, my brave friend.

Me: *Maybe. For sure, I'm in it to win it. But I can't do it alone.*

Jesus' followers are called his body. His precious, broken body. Everyone matters in the body of believers; without one another we're incomplete. I couldn't make it through cancer without people like my husband, who has been there for every single chemo session. I'm boosted by others who have helped carry my load. They're the living body of Christ, here and now. Each word and act of kindness speaks to my heart. That shouldn't be surprising since it's closer to the surface now.

All will be well.

WONDERFULLY MADE

Where can I go from your Spirit?
Where can I flee from your presence?

—PSALM 139:7, NIV

Me: *Can't wait to sink my toes in the sand.*

Marilyn: *It's here, waiting for you!*

My twin sister and I strolled Rehoboth's boardwalk together under circling gulls and heavy clouds. I clutched my flowered head scarf, hoping my wig underneath wouldn't blow into the sea. It was my first morning in Delaware, skipping chemo for a week—with my oncologist's stamp of approval—to be a beach bum. "Quality of life is important too," he had said, so off I trotted with visions of naps under a shady umbrella. I needed an umbrella, all right. Storms drenched my plans. While Jim fished in the rain, I hunkered down indoors with a novel.

Lewes, Delaware, where Marilyn lives, is along a major route for migrating birds. Jim and I, new at birding, were eager to see flocks heading south. No such luck. Wind and rain persisted. We slipped in a single outing when our daughter Julie and her husband, Bob, visited over a weekend. Trekking along Gordon's Pond at Cape Henlopen State Park, we spotted a gray heron, an osprey, and other waterfowl I couldn't identify. I climbed a platform and gazed across the pond through my monocular. Nope, no idea what was flapping around out there. Julie simply enjoyed the view, pointing out that one needn't know the names of the birds to appreciate their beauty. Then we hiked over dunes to an empty beach. The breeze was so gentle that my pink ball cap stayed in place. The surf washed over my bare feet, and sunshine warmed my skin. When there is but a single hour of sun in a week, its light is magnified.

One stormy morning, Marilyn and her husband, Jim, invited my Jim and me to their neighborhood prayer group called PUSH (Pray Until Something Happens). Our hostess, Donna, said her favorite psalm is 139. It's mine too. Hesitantly, I shared with this group of strangers a verse imprinted on my soul: "I praise you because I am fearfully and wonderfully made; your works are wonderful, I know that full well" (Ps. 139:14, NIV). Our hostess smiled as our eyes connected across the room. She said she'd read those very words in her morning devotions. Coincidence? Or, more likely, God-incidence. The Spirit first spoke to me through this psalm during my final pregnancy, assuring me that God's eyes were on my unborn baby. She's the strong, agile young woman who hiked with us at Gordon's Pond.

In between raindrops, my sister and I visited the labyrinth at old St. Peter's Episcopal Church in Lewes. Walking a stone-lined path where someone else stepped before me was a reminder that others have led the way through cancer's convoluted maze. We never walk alone. God is intimately acquainted with us. There's no hiding from the depths of this kind of love.

"How precious to me are your thoughts, God! How vast is the sum of them! Were I to count them, they would outnumber the grains of sand—when I awake, I am still with you" (Ps. 139:17-18, NIV).

All will be well.

The Practice of Walking a Labyrinth

Thus says the LORD:
Stand at the crossroads, and look,
and ask for the ancient paths,
where the good way lies; and walk in it,
and find rest for your souls.

—JEREMIAH 6:16

Unlike some spiritual practices, walking a labyrinth gets us on our feet. A labyrinth is a space designed with a path leading to a center and out again, offering a haven and a challenge. A large one can look intimidating until we start it. Then it sends oxygen to lungs, brain, and heart; quiets pesky interior chatter; and invites us to follow where earlier seekers have walked and prayed. There is an invisible chain of pilgrims going back to the first church labyrinth in Rome, created to encourage unbelievers and believers alike to ponder the holy mysteries of newly sanctioned Christianity. For some, it may have represented a pilgrimage to the holy city of Jerusalem.

Step by step, prayer by prayer, I find my inner self settling as I travel a labyrinth. I usually become more aware of God's presence along the way, but sometimes the world intrudes on this peaceful activity. It happened on a ninety-degree day under the scorching sun when gnats swarmed me at Bethany, a beautiful

Roman Catholic retreat center in rural Pennsylvania, proving no spiritual practice is without its vexations. Like life, a labyrinth isn't about reaching a goal as much as it is about each small step taken along the way.

A sign at the labyrinth outside St. Peter's Episcopal Church in Lewes, Delaware, says it is "A Path of Peace for all." A church brochure adds, "There is no right or wrong way to walk the Labyrinth. With only one path in, take it and you will arrive at the center. You may want to take a deep breath and focus on an intention as you walk."[8]

Once, when I walked a rustic, wooded path in Princeton, New Jersey, I was grateful it was a labyrinth, not a maze. A maze is confusing; just the thought of one causes my heart to race. A labyrinth does just the opposite.

My Celtic pilgrimage roommate, Judy, visited Ireland again after my diagnosis of breast cancer, where she walked the labyrinth at Glendalough on my behalf with Fr. Michael Rodgers, the mystic who lives there. What a lovely way to honor a friend. Maybe there is someone in your life you might offer up to God while walking a labyrinth.

Another option is a finger labyrinth. If you've never walked a labyrinth and are looking for moments of undistracted calm, finger labyrinth designs can be found online. Print a design of one that speaks to you. Sit in a quiet space and move your finger slowly along its symbolic path. If used repetitively during time set aside for meditation, a finger labyrinth is relaxing and quiets the soul.

Whether you walk with your feet or your fingers, labyrinths offer a centering activity for your soul. Give it a try the next time you're looking for a new spiritual practice.

***

Walking a labyrinth can be a way to practice mindfulness, thinking about the next spot to place your foot and living fully in the moment. You may feel uneasy the first time you walk a labyrinth. Just take your time and concentrate on each step, trusting that the way in really is the way out. No one gets lost in a labyrinth. It's a clearly defined path that leads to a center, providing a sacred place for contemplation. Find a labyrinth near you through the World-Wide Labyrinth Locator, an easy-to-use database (https:// labyrinthlocator.com). I live in rural western Pennsylvania and quickly found fourteen labyrinths within fifty miles of my home, most at churches or retreat centers.

REMEMBERING

"Very truly I tell you, unless a kernel of wheat
falls to the ground and dies, it remains only
a single seed. But if it dies, it produces
many seeds. Anyone who loves their life will
lose it, while anyone who hates their life in
this world will keep it for eternal life."

—JOHN 12:24-25, NIV

I came across a verse jotted in my mother's longhand:

> A haze on the far horizon,
> The infinite, tender sky,
> The ripe, rich tint of the cornfields,
> And the wild geese sailing high.
> And all over upland and lowland
> The charm of the golden-rod—
> Some of us call it Autumn
> 'And others call it God.'[9]

Born in 1919, Mother memorized poetry during her school
days in New Jersey. Later, as a young wife and Penn State student, she had her own radio show reading poems on the local
station. Imagine that happening today! My stay-at-home mom,
a *homemaker* in 1950s lingo, surprised my siblings and me by
learning to drive, returning to campus for education credits, and

beginning her career teaching English at forty. We entered junior high school together—Mother, Marilyn, and me. She stayed until we were moms ourselves.

In the background of my childhood is Mother's soprano voice. Sometimes she or Daddy played the upright piano. Sheet music was passed down from Grandpa Wesp, some of which is still in a box under my bed. Strains of the World War I song "My Buddy" filter through my thoughts each November: "Nights are long since you went away / I think about you all through the day . . . my buddy, my buddy, your buddy misses you."[10] Mother always sang "*somebody* misses you" because she had a special buddy in mind, an uncle she never met.

My mother's mother, Grandma Wesp, born in 1896, was orphaned by tuberculosis, both parents gone by the time she reached ten. My grandmother and her siblings went to live with their grandparents until they died. After that, she and her two young brothers set up housekeeping, as they called it, in West Hoboken, New Jersey. Her brother Fred lied about his age and enlisted in the Marines at seventeen. Within a year, he was killed in a foxhole in France. Grandma never fully recovered from that loss. Later, Uncle Bob told me how he survived the invasion of Normandy, D-Day, as a young pilot: "My mother lost a brother in the first war. I couldn't let her lose a son in the second."

Memories usually fade into black and white, but this one remains in vivid color. I see Grandma and me sitting on her plush teal-green bedroom carpet. She opened the bottom drawer of her secretary and pulled out a stack of letters Fred wrote from the war. We wept as she read aloud. "I didn't think I could still cry after all these years," she said, clutching them tightly.

***

"Death is a part of life," Mom said to me, after most of her generation was gone. We spoke openly of her own crossing over as the time grew near. Her Depression-era sense of practicality carried her through her losses.

"Someday you'll wake up and be in heaven, Mom," I whispered, my eyes misting.

"Won't that be wonderful!" Soothing my tears, she added, "Don't cry, dear. It's only natural."

Now that I'm living with cancer, I've returned to the wisdom of her words a thousand times. Mother folded into a smaller version of herself near the end of her ninety-one years, like a water lily at close of day. She left behind scraps of poetry stuck in books but knew how to release people, things, and ideas that might disrupt her sense of peace. She didn't know it by this name, but she was practicing the discipline of detachment. I'm still learning to do that. When I'm less attached, I feel less urgency to be judgmental, defensive, and anxious. Changing my thought patterns is hard work, and I'm not there yet. Cancer teaches patience, beginning with being patient with myself.

In honor of my mom's affection for poetry, I try my hand at a few lines, Celtic style:

> Praise you Father, Son and Spirit.
> Like the sun rising o'er the hills,
> I rise from last night's gloom.
> Alive to this fresh day,
> Still damp with possibilities.

Mom would like that.

All will be well.

SHAPING WORRIES INTO PRAYERS

"Though the mountains be shaken
and the hills be removed,
yet my unfailing love for you will not be shaken
nor my covenant of peace be removed,"
says the LORD, who has compassion on you.

—ISAIAH 54:10, NIV

I managed to keep my head on straight after hearing that a 7.8 earthquake on the Richter scale shook New Zealand, but my stomach churned at the thought of Tara's family living in a quake zone. When I looked online, I saw mini-quakes occurring practically every day.

Yikes! You put my family on that island, Lord?

The day after the first and most severe earthquake, Tara posted the following on Facebook:

> *Still rockin' and rattling here. There were two simultaneously—both rated "severe"—about ten minutes ago. Our bed is literally still swaying. I feel weirdly seasick.*
>
> **Me:** *Wrapping you in constant prayers. Hope they insulate you from harm.*

New Zealand was formed by volcanoes and is in an active earthquake zone called the Ring of Fire that encircles the Pacific. Though concerned for my family, I know I can't control nature. As a woman who likes to be in charge, I added another item to the list labeled, "Things Beyond My Control." Until now, cancer topped the list.

God pointed out I'm not in the driver's seat years ago when Tara and her husband, Derek, moved to North Philly. To this small-town girl, big-city Philadelphia was a scary place. In the way God arranges things, I happened to attend a media conference in the City of Brotherly Love before they moved into a spacious, three-story row home there.

I felt surprisingly at ease walking from our hotel to a neighborhood shop for breakfast with a friend, eating bagels under a cheerful sun umbrella our first morning at the conference. Little fissures in my fear crackled and spread with each step I took during breaks past Betty Ross' house, through Independence Hall, and down Broad Street. As my coworkers and I drove past the Museum of Art where Rocky raced up the steps, God seemed to smile and whisper, *Jan, you're not the Holy Spirit. You can't always be with your children. But I'm with them.* More icy anxiety melted in the warmth of God's heavenly wisdom.

In 2004, Tara and Derek invited Julie, who was eight years younger, to move in with them and attend Temple University. Today, Julie and her husband, Bob, own a century-old row home with pine floors and tall windows in South Philadelphia and claim the city as their own.

But New Zealand, Lord? That's another story!

Worry may be my native language, but the Word gives me a better way to talk: "Don't worry about anything, but pray about everything. With thankful hearts offer up your prayers and requests to God. Then, because you belong to Christ Jesus, God will bless you with peace that no one can completely understand. And this peace will control the way you think and feel" (Phil. 4:6-7, CEV).

It takes practice to release worries. It's easy to feel paralyzed when fearful shadows fall. Instead, I choose to ask, "Where's the light in this place?" It can be as close as the nearest window. Light banishes darkness, like pulling up shades in the morning. Saint Paul wrote this to new believers: "You are all children of light and children of the day; we are not of the night or of darkness" (1 Thess. 5:5).

I live with cancer. My family lives in a faraway earthquake zone. And I live as a daughter of the day, resting on the rock of God's unshakable goodness.

All will be well.

BELOVED

The LORD is my strength and my shield;
my heart trusts in him, and he helps me.
My heart leaps for joy,
and with my song I praise him.

—PSALM 28:7, NIV

I'm on a new chemo regimen, and—Alleluia!—my hair is growing back earlier than I expected. It's peach fuzz, but hey, I'll take it. In a rush of happiness, I shampooed and conditioned all half-inch of it, singing in the shower, "O come, all ye thankful."

Wait. That's wrong.

It's "all ye *faithful*," not "all ye *thankful*."

Chemo brain. Garbled speech, confused thinking, fuzzy facts, names just beyond reach. Evidently, I was thinking (using that word loosely) of "Come, Ye Thankful People, Come." Both songs are from an era when English-speaking folks said *ye* and *thee* a lot more than we do. Both are sung to celebrate holidays that arrive as bitter winds blow the Northern Hemisphere into winter. Both invite us to move closer together for human and divine warmth, to gather in community as part of something bigger than ourselves.

"O come, all ye faithful, joyful and triumphant, O come ye, O come ye to Bethlehem."

In the 1700s, German and French monks sang "Adeste Fideles" ("O Come, All Ye Faithful") on the holiest of nights.

The melody takes me back to Christmas Eve in my home church, with robed choirs proceeding down the aisle, my kids in miniature robes among them. Chemo causes memory lapses, but it can't steal this one. While waiting for the brain fog to clear, I'm thankful for small things, like laughter. Hair. My husband, who does chores I never notice. Christmas and a tree with ornaments to hang, each with a unique history, however dim my memory may be.

Along with gray matter, my energy is still missing. My legs wobble if I walk to the end of the street. I'm thankful the ancient carol doesn't say, "O come, all ye useful." As a Christian, Christmas declares I'm inherently beloved, regardless of what I can or cannot do, my résumé, or my cluttered pile of weaknesses. At the core of my existence, I was created for undying friendship with the One who came as a baby in Bethlehem. We all were. My identity isn't tied to what I do. It's relentlessly bound up in the essence of who I am and whose I am. It's like I'm wearing new glasses that are finally in focus, allowing me to see everyone on the globe as God's beloved, beginning with the person I see in the mirror.

Janet, a Ugandan mother who shares my name and breast cancer: *Indeed, all will be well!*

Six months ago, I marked and dated this passage in my Bible: "There is a river whose streams make glad the city of God, the holy place where the Most High dwells. God is within her, she will not fall; God will help her at break of day" (Ps. 46:4-5, NIV). Today, I plunge again into its strength. I pause and breathe in the wonder of worshiping Jesus.

God is with me, muddled mind and all. Call me a kid, but this old girl is counting down the days to my final chemotherapy session and the moment the last drop drips through my port. It's a Christmas morning kind of feeling.

"O come, let us adore him"!

All will be well.

RESOUNDING JOY

Let the sea resound, and everything in it,
the world, and all who live in it.
Let the rivers clap their hands,
let the mountains sing together for joy.

—PSALM 98:7-8, NIV

Julie was in first grade when her music teacher telephoned to say our youngest child knew every word of every carol. "How can that be?" she asked. The teacher's question surprised me. How was Julie's knowledge anything but ordinary? Playing and singing carols is a tradition at our house. We kick off the season the first day it snows, often with Bert Kaempfert's instrumental version of "Sleigh Ride"—even if it's October (and it usually is). Bells ringing automatically shifts me into Christmas mode. But not this time. Jim put on "Joy to the World," and I cried.

Fatigue's gray cloud of irritation weighs me down. As much as silence calms me, maybe it's time to bang some pots and pans and make some holy clamor. Psalm 98:4 says, "Shout for joy to the LORD, all the earth, burst into jubilant song with music" (NIV). This very psalm inspired Isaac Watts to write "Joy to the World" in 1791. Watts described nature's voice roaring praises to the Creator: "While fields and floods, rocks, hills, and plains, repeat the sounding joy." O Lord, do I listen closely enough to hear fields and floods singing their love for you? Help me praise you like the hills and rocks do!

Joining nature's praise choir, despite my gray mood, would put me in good company. Small rituals add meaning too. When our kids were young, we lit the candles of an Advent wreath each Sunday. With my energy duller than a string of burnt-out twinkle lights, Jim and I are trying a simpler ritual. In the Celtic Christian tradition, we're lighting a single candle for forty nights, seeking God's benediction on each day. A candle testifies to the Lord's flickering, persistent light within me, regardless of how I feel.

Jesus understands my dullness of heart but refuses to let it keep me from his table. I may feel disconnected from the Lord on occasion, but God never tires of waiting for me. The entire Trinity invites me inside the circle of God's divine love. One draws me close. One blankets me in comfort. Another goes to a cross and back on my behalf. May this season remind us of the "wonder of [God's] love."

All will be well.

The Practice of Lament

With a loud cry, Jesus breathed his last.

—MARK 15:37, NIV

I felt unequal to the weight of describing this practice until hospital tests came back with troubling results. Then I opened the book of Lamentations and read Jeremiah's funeral dirge for Israel, grieving for sinful people who had lost everything. I grieve for my family if I die, understanding when Jeremiah says, "See, O LORD, how distressed I am; my stomach churns, my heart is wrung within me" (Lam. 1:20). When he mourns, "Joy is gone from our hearts; our dancing has turned to mourning" (Lam. 5:15, NIV), my soul cries, "I'm with you, brother!"

Christmas, in particular, can be steeped in sadness and sorrow. We may be grieving a loss, be encumbered by a broken relationship, or be aching with that undefinable, universal pang of isolation and longing that is part of being human. Some churches recognize that the language of lament has an authentic place in Advent by offering "Longest Night" services at the time of the winter solstice, tying inner shadows to outer darkness. We sometimes forget there was lamenting that first Christmas when Herod decreed the murder of Jewish baby boys in the small village of Bethlehem. While angels were singing, a paranoid king was plotting the massacre of innocent children, memorialized in the Feast of the Innocents in Catholic and Byzantine churches. In our world, where violence happens daily, it's more than fitting to respond with tears and anguish. In Western culture, most lamenting is done privately, not communally; but beyond personal loss, we grieve human suffering, injustice, and environmental havoc. Advocating against the sale of assault weapons and for better mental health services are examples of ways to let communal loss spur us on to positive action.

If we live long enough, we all have reasons to practice lament as a spiritual discipline. If you're sorrowing, please know Jesus entered into humanity to identify with you and enter into the distress you feel at this very moment. When you are desolate, know the angels of heaven encompass you in prayer. I told my grieving neighbor the day after her husband died that I'd have faith for her when she could not. It's compelling that laments in scripture are addressed to God. Prophets and psalmists wailed, "How long must suffering continue?" These people trusted mighty God enough to know they wouldn't be rejected if they kept it real.

It is hard to continue when our days are eclipsed by tears, but the Word tells us death doesn't have the final word. "But we do not want you to be uninformed, brothers and sisters, about those who have died, so that you may not grieve as others do who have no hope" (1 Thess. 4:13).

In the midst of despair like Jeremiah's, we catch glimpses of grace:

> This I call to mind,
>> and therefore I have hope:
> The steadfast love of the LORD never ceases,
>> his mercies never come to an end;
> they are new every morning;
>> great is your faithfulness.
> "The LORD is my portion," says my soul,
>> "therefore I will hope in him." (Lam. 3:21-24)

When we recognize lament as a biblical and historical practice, we give ourselves and others permission to do it, shadowing in our own small way Jesus' sense of abandonment on the cross when he cried, "My God, my God, why have you forsaken me?" (Matt. 27:46).

***

According to Merriam-Webster, *lamentation* can be defined as an "expression of sorrow, mourning, or regret." As a spiritual practice, lament provides an intentional way to face unbearable agony, all the while crying out to God for help. Study Lamentations 1:1-4, and try this exercise from *The Spiritual Formation Bible*: "After reading these verses, remember a time you felt absolutely alone and defeated. Write your own description of that anguished point in your life. Feel free to make parallels to the scripture verses. Try to use vivid language as you detail the rejection and hopelessness you felt. Read your 'lamentation' aloud and offer your words to the God who has never left you, even when you felt alone."[11]

(Lament is a normal expression of grief; ongoing depression is not. If you're experiencing sadness that causes you concern for your mental health or safety, or that of others, please seek medical help.)

HALFWAY THROUGH THE DARK

Even the darkness is not dark to You,
And the night is as bright as the day.
Darkness and light are alike *to You.*

—PSALM 139:12, NASB

There he was, a little guy wearing a Steelers ball cap and a grin, standing in the sanctuary doorway. Yes, we're both Pittsburgh Steelers fans, but we have more in common than that. So full of spunk with that great smile—how could *he* have cancer? His mama introduced Andrew and herself, saying she reads bits of my column to him. Only eight, he understands a battle that no child should have to. I knelt down to shake his hand, and his smile told me I was going to love this kid. We hugged. Andrew's hair was missing, but his complexion announced he was a ginger, like my Irish ancestors and youngest daughter, Julie. Cancer feels like somebody punched out all the stars, leaving black holes where light belongs. Andrew's parents know that feeling far too well. Yet cancer pushes me to seek pinpoints of hope where light seeps through. Hope anchors me to the steadfastness of God.

I think of Stone Age astronomers who studied the stars. Among them were prehistoric people in Ireland who built an acre-size mound today called Newgrange. It held a secret deep within its burial tomb for more than a thousand years. On our

Irish pilgrimage, friends and I squeezed through a narrow passageway leading to its dark innermost chamber. We emerged in silent awe, squinting in the light.

Newgrange took generations to construct, beginning a thousand years before work began on Stonehenge. The tomb eventually fell into ruin until road builders rediscovered it in 1699. Excavation began centuries later, in the early 1960s. A few years later a roof box was uncovered. When debris was cleared, archaeologists discovered that for exactly seventeen minutes at dawn on the winter solstice, a beam of light penetrates through that little box, down the narrow interior passage and into the cross-shaped chamber. Like a massive sundial, Newgrange tracks light.

Winter's arrival means we're halfway through the dark. Celebrating this astronomical event in late December with captured sunlight took wisdom and ingenuity. Like the magi, these ancients were guided by stars.

* * *

I sent a craft package with old maps tucked inside for my grand-boys to make Christmas stars after I saw a tree, covered with them.

Tara: Love the map stars!

Me: A way of connecting with something beyond the here and now...

And a way to stay connected with our boys, who now view the Southern Hemisphere's night sky with its different constellations. Despite years of chemo ahead that lower his immunity and increase his risk of catching germs, Andrew may soon return to school, ice hockey, and happier times, like my grandchildren experience. If prehistoric astronomers could design Newgrange, still an accurate timepiece after five thousand years, researchers today must have equal determination to cure childhood cancer.

Chemotherapy is over for me, at least for now. Hope is like a small shaft of light on the darkest night of the year. I begin thirty-six radiation sessions in the new year. In a remarkable pair of verses, Psalm 147:3-4 (NIV), God ministers to us with one hand and paints a heavenly tableau with the other: "He heals the broken-hearted and binds up their wounds. He determines the number of the stars and calls them each by name."

All will be well.

HUMILITY'S DOOR

What, then, shall we say in response to these things? If God is for us, who can be against us? He who did not spare his own Son, but gave him up for us all—how will he not also, along with him, graciously give us all things?

—ROMANS 8:31-32, NIV

There is a small doorway in Bethlehem called the "Door of Humility." I had to bow low to enter this traditional site of Christ's birth, while children are small enough to run right in, as if their father owns the place. The doorway to the massive stone Church of the Nativity is only about four feet high and half as wide; the top lintel was lowered to stop looters and invaders on horseback from trampling through the holy site. It leads to a dim basilica, lined with limestone pillars. I shivered and pulled my jacket close, thinking how bleak the cave below must have felt when Mary and Joseph bedded down with cattle, waiting for her baby to be born.

In 1868, Episcopal preacher Phillips Brooks wrote "O Little Town of Bethlehem" to help the children in his congregation better understand what happened that holy night.[12] Brooks probably told them first about riding on horseback one Christmas Eve across the famed Shepherds' Fields and then worshiping with crowds in the Church of the Nativity. Then Brooks introduced the children to a new Christmas hymn. After he wrote the lyrics, he asked the church organist, Lewis H. Redner, to compose a tune. Redner noted that "It was after midnight that a little angel whispered the strain in my ears, and I roused myself and jotted it down as you have it."[13]

When I read the history of this carol, I thought of treading down narrow stairs to the cave below the basilica, to the traditional spot of Jesus' birth. Of singing of the little town with friends in that damp nook. Of the sprawling place where it all began, lined with noisy streets where Palestinian children now play. How the world aches for the Christ child!

Christmas means more than ever to me this year. I've been brought down by the gravity of breast cancer cells invading my body, like unruly horsemen prancing into a sanctuary. I've stooped low before God and circumstances as I await health's return. After struggling through difficult emotions with each new challenge, I remember who I am—God's daughter, led by the sure hand of my Father. I begin radiation therapy Tuesday. With chemo behind me, I posted this on Facebook:

> **Me:** *That's done!*
>
> **Friend:** *Cue the heavenly chorus!*
>
> **Me:** *Amen!*

I carry burdens into this Christmas, but my spirit and feet were created to run into God's presence. Why do I settle for less? God sent the Son to earth as a child. That humble way is the only way to come. Jesus said, "Let the little ones come to me, don't ever stop a one of them! Heaven's kingdom belongs to people exactly like them" (Matt. 19:14, AP).

Friend Claudia: *I began to feel stressed as I pondered the time we devote to the craziness of the secular side of Christmas—so many expectations and activities to fill our lives when I just want to focus my heart and center it on the birth of our Savior. Joy to the world, the Lord has come!*

Me: *I so often feel like this, Claudia. Joy to the world, the Lord has come!*

Here is part of a little-known last verse of "O Little Town of Bethlehem" that moved me:

> Where charity stands watching
> And faith holds wide the door,
> The dark night wakes, the glory breaks,
> And Christmas comes once more.[14]

Sometimes doors slam shut. One did in Bethlehem. A baby boy was born that night anyhow. His birth in a low cave made it sacred. Jesus' birth in you and me transforms us into sanctuaries of his Spirit.

All will be well.

GOD IS

The LORD your God is God of gods and Lord of
lords, the great God, mighty and awesome,
who shows no partiality and accepts no bribes.

—DEUTERONOMY 10:17, NIV

One day, Fiona knocked on our door. Smiling, she handed me
a book. Her own. "Here's my book, Grandma!" She titled it *40
Days to Reflect on Your Walk with the Lord.*[15] I had happily encour-
aged her but was still astonished to actually see it in print. Holding Fiona's book in my hands, I resolved to finally write my own,
my goal for the year. If she could do it at eighteen, why can't I do
it later in life?

To refresh my skills and prove to myself I was serious, I
enrolled in an online writing course. Then life happened. Suddenly, cancer demanded all my attention. This is why resolutions
get a bad rap. Life comes along and messes with our best intentions. I didn't get far with the course or the book, but I began
telling my story every week in the newspaper. My resolve to write
was reconfigured by my circumstances.

Instead of making resolutions, for years I've prayed John
Wesley's Covenant Prayer, a New Year's tradition among Meth-
odists for more than 250 years. A covenant is an agreement
between partners, like marriage vows. Wesley's prayer requires
me to lay down my hopes, desires, and expectations—a far jump

from New Year's resolutions—and toss my lot totally into God's hands. It reads:

> I am no longer my own, but thine.
> Put me to what thou wilt, rank me with whom
>   thou wilt.
> Put me to doing, put me to suffering.
> Let me be employed by thee or laid aside for thee,
> exalted for thee or brought low for thee.
> Let me be full, let me be empty.
> Let me have all things, let me have nothing.
> I freely and heartily yield all things
> to thy pleasure and disposal. (UMH, no. 607)

How do I possibly live this out? Very imperfectly. My spirit is attentive, but my mind is like a willow in the wind. Peace comes in practicing my breath prayer and in trusting the Sacred Three to equip me to do what I'm called to do. I get the feeling Wesley knew them intimately, for he closed his prayer saying:

> And now, O Glorious and blessed God,
> Father, Son, and Holy Spirit,
> thou art mine, and I am thine. So be it.
> And the covenant which I have made on earth,
> Let it be ratified in heaven. Amen. (UMH, no. 607)

God empowers me to keep my promise as I lean on my Keeper (see Psalm 121:5), like the old prophet Zechariah: "'Not by might, nor by power, but by my spirit, says the LORD of hosts'" (Zech. 4:6). He knew the Lord of heavenly armies had his back, and I do too. An unseen army of God's angels surrounds me as I begin radiation treatments. A friend said during her sessions that she pictured Jesus as the fourth man in the fiery furnace protecting her. Another one silently recited the Lord's Prayer three times each trip through the radiation clinic. By the time she was done, her treatment was too.

Wesley's prayer may sound too old-school or just plain overwhelming. I'm praying breath prayers during radiation—inhaling with "God" and slowly exhaling "is."

God is. God is. God is.

Knowing the great I Am is as close as my breath calms my jitters, relaxes my body, releases my worries, corrals my scattered thoughts.

God is.

I learned that prayer in Glendalough, where God's presence seems to seep like mist from Irish mountains, lakes, and monastic ruins. In an ancient cemetery, I was taught a simple affirmation by the resident mystic: "I am. Things are. God is." Do I really need to know anything beyond this?

I am. Things are. God is. Amen.

> **Rebecca, whose son Andrew who is recovering from leukemia:** Just read your column and I have to tell you I'll be using "God is." Andrew recently had two trips to the ER due to fevers. Those were four hard days! I wish that I'd had "God is." I'll be using it every time his care becomes overwhelming.*

All will be well.

---

* Andrew is now healthy, in school, involved in sports, and an acolyte at church.

The Practice of Breath Prayer

"Whenever you pray, go into your room and shut
the door and pray to your Father who is in secret;
and your Father who sees in secret will reward you."

—MATTHEW 6:6

It's meaningful to join in a practice that unites us with millions of other Christians. For at least fifteen hundred years, Orthodox believers have offered this breath prayer: "Lord Jesus Christ, Son of God, have mercy on me, a sinner." Known as the Jesus Prayer, it can be whispered in a single breath. Today's condensed form, used by Christians of many persuasions, is this: "Lord Jesus Christ, Son of God, have mercy."

From a baby's first cry to our final breath, breathing is the most natural and essential thing we do. Relating prayer to intentional breathing makes us more aware of both. I started praying this way while meeting with friends regularly to practice Centering Prayer. By candlelight, we silently contemplate our own prayer for twenty minutes. For years, mine was simply "Jesus."

I increased my devotion to breath prayers after being diagnosed with cancer and taking up yoga. I now pause for a few moments of controlled breathing throughout the day, especially when stressed. My yoga instructor taught us four steps for each breath: slowly breathe in; hold still for a moment; slowly breathe out; and again, briefly hold still.

Since my pilgrimage to Ireland, my breath prayer has changed to "God" (inhale) "is" (exhale). The shorter the prayer, the easier it is for my brain to stay centered. These can be entirely wordless prayers at times, expressing a sense that we are vessels of God's Spirit. (See "The Practice of Sacramental Living.") Just as Jesus turned water into wine at a wedding party, Jesus breathes life into our breath prayers. In my blog, I wrote of relying on my breath prayer in an anxious moment: "A wily foe sneaks in, as often happens when I attempt to snooze. Anxiety gnaws at my innards, spreading cold apprehension. My eyes are too heavy to open, but I practice measured breathing, repeating my breath prayer: God is. My torso swells and relaxes, gentle as last summer's waves at Lewes Beach. Worry's power to disrupt my rest is washed away."

Practicing controlled breathing is one of the most sacred things we can do, acknowledging that the Spirit is in this and every moment. As Jesus reminds us in John 6:63, "It is the spirit that gives life." Breath prayer is a simple way to pray, trusting God to know all the details, all the troubles, all the complexities and hopes contained there.

***

Breath prayer synchronizes our bodily rhythm with our awareness of the presence of God and reminds us that praying is as necessary as breathing. We can practice breath prayers any time or place, alone or in a crowd. Try it when you need to stay calm or focused or to help you listen more intently as a loved one shares her concerns. While increasing your attentiveness to your surroundings, these little prayers put the brain and soul in gear, helping you tune in to the leading of God's Spirit.

GOD'S SONG

The LORD, your God, is in your midst,
a warrior who gives victory;
he will rejoice over you with gladness,
he will renew you in his love;
he will exult over you with loud singing.

—ZEPHANIAH 3:17

In December, weary from facing down cancer, Jim and I visited Pittsburgh's Phipps Conservatory and Botanical Gardens. We welcomed the change of scenery, meandering through the century-old glasshouse, past antique sleighs and thousands of poinsettias. Sipping cocoa to stay warm, I tucked my scarf deeper into a red wool jacket, thankful to be alive. Thankful for fuzz on my shiny head. Thankful to be surrounded by strangers and their kids, skipping around a fantasy crystal lake. A fantasy night for me.

Earlier Jim and I had stopped by a holiday gathering at the seminary where I studied spiritual formation. Two women and I munched cookies together and discovered we'd all survived breast cancer. Both of these women are ordained, a fact that reminded me faith isn't a magic wand shielding believers from the risky task of being human.

Friends had offered Jim and me the use of their studio apartment for the night. In the morning, we strolled through the neighborhood of Victorian homes to Commonplace Coffee, where we ran into hometown friends. Over muffins, they introduced us to yet another cancer survivor. Her story and the stories of others help me trust that my own will someday be ancient history too. More than that, I trust that God hovers near, singing goodness into my days and nights.

Later, while walking in a nearby park, I noticed "Joy is an act of resistance" scrolled in a metal garden gate. It reminded me to choose tenacious joy, no matter what. My joy isn't locked away, accessible only when grand things happen in my life. I find it in simple activities of everyday life, such as folding laundry, sending a note to a friend, listening to grandsons Eli and Josiah giggle on the phone.

After our getaway weekend, I froze through my final chemotherapy treatment, once again holding ice in gloved hands to fight neuropathy. Sometimes during chemo, I'd close my eyes and think of God singing over everyone hooked up to machines in that room. Psalm 42:8 says, "The LORD will send His goodness in the daytime; and His song will be with me in the night, A prayer to the God of my life" (NASB).

Psalm 42:8 echoes my "life verse," which I turn to again and again. Sometimes I read my life verse in a variety of translations to catch more of God's song:

> "The LORD your God is in your midst,
> A victorious warrior.
> He will rejoice over you with joy,
> He will be quiet in His love,
> He will rejoice over you with shouts of joy."
> (Zeph. 3:17, NASB)

A breast cancer survivor gave me a bracelet of smooth purple stones. It has a heart-shaped locket she wore during her radiation sessions. Afterward, we messaged each other:

Breast cancer survivor: Tuck a thought inside the locket and wear it to radiation.

Me to survivor: I put my life verse inside.

Day or night, chemo or radiation, whether I'm feeling strong or down, God's love song is always in the background, like Mother's voice in my childhood. I might not hear it, it might be muffled by noisy clutter, or I may choose to tune it out. But God's song— a song of hope and redemption—fills more than choir lofts. It resounds through all eternity. How sweet the sound.

All will be well.

WINGED BLESSINGS

"Ask the animals, and they will teach you,
or the birds in the sky, and they will tell you;
or speak to the earth, and it will teach you,
or let the fish in the sea inform you.
Which of all these does not know
that the hand of the LORD has done this?"

—JOB 12:7-9, NIV

Call it the communion of saints, heavenly nudges, or bits of whimsy. God is sending me cardinals—splashes of color against the dull winter sky. Not only bright males but a tawny female too, wearing hints of red, her feathers plumped for warmth. Marilyn started this cardinal business after my mastectomy, asking Mom to send me one. Within five minutes, a bright-red fellow appeared on the deck. Soon I was sharing these occurrences with others.

> **Me:** *Cardinals are my symbol of hope.*
>
> **Barbara:** *Love it! We have seven male cardinals that visit our feeders, all here this morning. Cardinals were my mom's favorites.*
>
> **Birder facing tough issues, who sees 'em by the dozen:** *I get God's "pick-me-ups" to keep me going on down days.*

I know what she means. I'm happy with my pair—serenading each other and checking out real estate for their first nest of the season while snow still blows. I picture them, twigs in beaks, chirping back and forth: "Do you like that branch better? Or does this one have a better view?" Perhaps they sing in the depths of winter because we need the promise of spring their voices foretell.

A hometown friend asks me if I've read Paula D'Arcy's book *Gift of the Red Bird: The Story of a Divine Encounter.* "The red bird becomes a symbol and reminder of God's presence," she tells me. In fact, I had ordered that very book moments before my friend's message arrived. Coincidence? Maybe more. I identified with D'Arcy's book; cancer can feel like the wilderness she experienced. Then I received Ronald Rolheiser's little volume from a friend, *Prayer: Our Deepest Longing.* The title says it all. Although our deepest longings can be masked by the busyness of a noisy culture, we know there is something more. It's so easy to forget that the Lord placed eternity in my heart. Eternity! (See Ecclesiastes 3:11, NASB.)

I glimpse life's wonder when I set aside distractions, seeking what's beneath the brittle surface of my days. Cancer frees me to let others run the world while I consider patterns of faithfulness in small things: birds, herbs, ferns. They teach me to trust the big stuff to their Maker, and mine.

Somebody said when you see a cardinal, angels are near.

Big Sis: *God's hand works in wonderful, mysterious ways. Angels indeed.*

Cardinals, swooping low to gather seed. Are they flashes of nature in flight or the rush of angel wings? Maybe both.

All will be well.

IRISH ADVENTURE

"I am the gate. Whoever enters by me will be saved, and will come in and go out.... I came that they may have life, and have it abundantly."

—JOHN 10:9-10

Saint Brigid's feast day is February first. It's easy for me to remember because it's my birthday. Midway between winter and spring, it is a celebration with roots far in the hazy past, as is Groundhog Day on February 2. Both mark the countdown to warmer, lighter days.

Is Brigid a woman of myth or history? My guess is a little of both. Ireland's female patron saint, she is revered for her generous hospitality. On my Celtic Christian pilgrimage, I stayed overnight in Kildare, her hometown. Sunny flower boxes and the aroma of warm bread from open windows greeted me, but it's a wee Irish adventure that unlocked something within me that I remember the most.

It was late afternoon when my group slipped into Kildare Cathedral, a magnificent, fenced-in stone church at the end of a downtown street. The guide, a woman wearing no-nonsense shoes and a proper skirt and blouse, announced it was almost closing time. My roommate, Judy, and I hurried through the interior and then, leaving our group, circled around back to a cemetery with Celtic crosses and a twelfth-century round tower. Everyone else was gone. The silence was calming until Judy said, "It's awfully quiet. I hope we're not locked in!"

Startled, I ran around front and down to the iron gate. A hefty chain secured it, guarded by imposing stone pillars. I resisted clinging to the bars of the gate (this was an adventure, right?), but my voice betrayed my jitters when I called to the only person in sight, a tourist on the street: "We're locked in here!" She hastened into a store. Moments later, a young shopkeeper appeared.

"If somebody's around, usually their car is here," the shopkeeper said doubtfully, pointing to an empty space as she approached a stone cottage and knocked. I exchanged glances with Judy, now by my side.

The door opened, and there was our guide. I blushed like a tardy schoolgirl. She strode toward us in her no-nonsense shoes as if she'd done this before and lifted the chain off the gate. "It's never locked," she said, her eyes meeting mine. Relieved, I pushed the heavy gate open. Somewhere, I think Saint Brigid smiled. We could have stood there for hours, assuming we were locked inside and unaware freedom was already ours. All we had to do was lift the chain.

When I feel trapped by fear—cancer's trademark—I look back on that afternoon and know things aren't always as they appear to be. For believers, freedom is a done deal. Sealed as soon as Jesus said those words from the cross, "It is finished." Walking in faith when I don't see the evidence—that's the tricky part.

In the shadows of the distant past, Saint Patrick, another Irish saint, tread through risky terrain, singing a *lorica* (prayer) of protection for his friends, his enemies, his God, and all the angels of heaven to hear. He took seriously Paul's admonition to "put on the full armor of God" (Eph. 6:11, NIV). His breastplate was goodness and honor, trusting Christ to be within him, behind him, before him, beside him. . . .[16]

* * *

During today's radiation treatment I lay on the table in semi-darkness, a disk gliding side to side over my bare chest. I shivered and wondered if every woman feels as vulnerable as I did at that moment, stripped before a couple of technicians, rays of radiation zooming toward targeted spots.

It was Father-daughter time, my way of detaching from an uncomfortable experience.

"My Word is a fiery sword," God whispered.

"You're my armor. My breastplate. My helmet. My peace," I answered. How can I ever forget you're in this with me, Lord?

I think of the radiation penetrating any remaining cancer cells as God's lightsaber, the stuff of vintage *Star Wars*. Our grandson Josiah draws superheroes, so I asked him to sketch a good guy rescuing me. I can see the word balloons now—"Bam!" "Smack!" "Outta here!" Goodbye, bad cells.

> **Friend:** *You remain in my heart and my soul. Thank you for sharing your continuous journey and faith.*

With the spirit of Saint Brigid's generous hospitality, I also glimpse another scene: that iron gate in Kildare, swung forever open because it's never locked. The One who offers us abundant life also sets us free: "If the Son sets you free, you will be free indeed" (John 8:36, NIV). God's heart is open and ready to welcome and comfort us, whatever we're facing.

All will be well.

The Practice of Pilgrimage

Blessed are those whose strength is in you,
whose hearts are set on pilgrimage.

—PSALM 84:5, NIV

For those with a searching soul, a pilgrimage can offer a unique way to connect with God. People who take up the challenge to travel into unfamiliar territory for a spiritual purpose often sense a call by God but may be uncertain why. *Pilgrimage* is rooted in the old French word *peligrinage*. A pilgrimage holds unexpected graces for the traveler open to unplanned possibilities. The destination can be as close as a downtown sanctuary or a wooded hillside, but usually it is to a new place—whether physically or mentally—that allows the pilgrim to see the world and the self in new light. The pilgrim's footsteps follow those who have gone before, although each person has a unique odyssey. (It took me a long time to become comfortable thinking of myself as a "pilgrim," unsure if I fit in with other dedicated faith travelers.)

On one of my pilgrimages, I found myself late one night at Prayer Mountain in South Korea, a stone's throw from the demilitarized zone (DMZ), I slipped out of bed, grabbed my flashlight, and made my way to a tiny, barren cubicle on an upper floor of the church beside our lodge. It was there for women (others were for men) to pray, with only a prayer rug and a light bulb hanging on a cord. As soon as I entered, I felt a great burden to kneel and lift up Korean mothers, daughters, and wives who knelt there before and after me. The next day I knelt for a moment in the DMZ, assured that prayer was why God had me there. I was blessed by those opportunities.

Pilgrimages also can involve formidable obstacles and challenges to reach a holy destination, like barefoot pilgrims who climb the rocky path up Croagh Patrick in Ireland. My longest pilgrimage is a metaphorical one, traveling the peaks, plains, and valleys of living with cancer.

A pilgrimage requires thoughtful spiritual and practical preparation; it is a good idea to read about the destination beforehand. Consider stretching yourself and your faith by stepping into unknown terrain. Perhaps a pilgrimage might be what you need to gain a fresh perspective—and surprising blessings.

* * *

Not all of us can take off to visit lands far and wide for a pilgrimage. But you can still experience the effect of transporting yourself from your current location to another environment through guided meditation. Call to mind a favorite place you like to visit, or maybe imagine a trip you've dreamed of taking. Concentrate on what you see. What does the scenery look like? Are there any sounds or smells to be noticed? What do you hear? Pay attention to where your soul guides you as you immerse yourself in another place and time. What is God saying to you there?

LOVE LETTER

Whoever does not love does not know God,
for God is love.

—1 JOHN 4:8

Here I am—flat on a table, pillow between my knees, eyes closed, hands clasped overhead. Those dim moments of daily radiation provide fifteen minutes of stillness. If I've rushed in, barely beating the clock, it's harder to reduce inner static. Praying my breath prayer, "God is," on day thirteen of thirty-six, I breathed *God is,* and it evolved into *God is patient. God is kind. God is love.*

A memory seeps through time.

I was in my ninth-grade science class, located in the school's basement, seated at a table with my only close friend beside me. We both ached with teenage angst that distracted us from whatever the teacher was talking about. Six words are all I recall from science that year.

"What is God?"

Her whisper caught me off guard. I paused, then said, "God is . . . love."

I don't remember anyone teaching me this. It simply rose from a deeper source of wisdom than was mine at age fifteen. (Later, in high school, I began reading the Bible and noticed John, the friend of Jesus, wrote those same words.) Something shifted in my center with her question. Still a lonely, skinny, flat-chested bookworm, I came to know that God would somehow use me to reach out to people who feel like nobodies—seeing them as somebodies with aches and hopes like mine. My girl-friend and I had many God-talks after that, and our conversation awakened a fragile sense of self-worth within me.

Three decades later, this friend traveled to our home for an overnight stay.

"I didn't know people really did that," she said, after Jim asked a blessing on our supper. "I thought it was only on TV!"

She said she felt pressured to measure up to others' expecta-tions growing up, never knowing love without strings attached. We talked more the next morning, until she was about to pull out of the driveway. Jim and I walked to her car, and I said, "Just remember—there's nothing you'll ever do to make God love you more. And you could never do anything to make God love you less. You're loved, just the way you are." She drove away shaking her head, as if I'd said red was green. But she was smiling.

Crazy, upside-down, inside-out, love-without-limits.

Conditional acceptance says, "If this, then that." Fickle as petal-picking a daisy. But unlimited love has no walls to climb, no tests to pass. Saint Paul wrote to nitpicky church people to say they could give away all they owned, understand every mystery in heaven and on earth, and have mountain-moving faith, but without love, it counted for nothing. Nada. Zilch. Nothing we do matters if it is not motivated by God's love. First Corinthians 13:7 attempts to paint love's infinite stretch: "It bears all things, believes all things, hopes all things, endures all things."

I put a question on Facebook, wondering how others define enduring love. The response closest to my heart was posted by a childhood friend:

What is love? I think, first, commitment.

Exactly. Commitment is a hefty concept that demands our all if we take it seriously. The woman who wrote that message read my mind. Love is commitment in action. I see it every day through this cancer drama. Jim, my leading man, fulfills a vow he made when all our days still lay before us, "For better or worse, for richer or poorer, in sickness and in health." Ours isn't a cheap paperback romance. It's a love that prepares meatloaf and repairs what's broken. Washes dishes. Chops firewood. Cleans toilets. Holds my hand in the dark. Committed love never gives up.

Whoever and wherever we are, lying on a beach or a radiation table, receiving Communion or a prison sentence, making peace or causing chaos, God's love is there too.

All will be well.

A TIME FOR WEEPING

Rouse yourself! Why do you sleep, O Lord?
Awake, do not cast us off forever!
Why do you hide your face?
Why do you forget our affliction and oppression?

—PSALM 44:23-24

Whoever wrote Psalm 44 was acquainted with the helplessness reeling through me after learning another friend died from cancer. *She trusted you, Lord. We all prayed, trusting you too! Where are you, God?*

Early in my cancer ordeal I heard from a young woman with ovarian cancer who was fighting with every fiber of her being to be there for her family. She was incredulous that I would consider skipping chemotherapy. After braving fifty chemo treatments, she couldn't conceive of anything less. On her Facebook page, she quoted Philippians 4:13: "I can do all things through him who strengthens me." I read of her death online while watching the Grammys, but after reading the news, I quickly turned off the TV. I needed time to lament.

Scripture provides a safe refuge to cry out unflinchingly to God. The psalmists ask hard questions. Sackcloth and ashes tell us Hebrew nomads knew the smell of death far too well. Today, we hide mourning behind sunglasses and closed doors, but if I put on a happy face right now, I'd be as fake as Hollywood makeup.

In the midst of agonizing losses, some words offered with good intentions fail to comfort a mourning heart. During my cancer journey, I've heard stuff like, "Praise God, who knows best." Or "It's best not to question God." And "God gave you this to make you stronger." And worse, "God needed so-and-so in heaven to be another angel."

Please!

I'd rather get wordless hugs than religious clichés. When I'm feeling weaker than a rag doll or mourning the loss of a valiant fighter, I don't feel like praising God. What I appreciate is the warmth of a friend's silent support when she walks arm in arm with me through sorrow's corridors.

Perhaps God's arms are open to embrace it all—our hurts, our questions, and the raw sense of betrayal when young kids lose their mom. I feel like beating God's chest and asking where the heck is love in this. It won't drive God away. God is big enough to take our grief and turn it into prayer. Even Jesus lamented and grieved. A crucifix tells me the wounds in Jesus' hands and feet are real. An empty cross says nails couldn't hold him. The full arc of Christ's journey—from manger to cross to resurrection—encourages me to move inch by inch, like a barefoot pilgrim on jagged rock, toward healing. The path is worn by others who braved the way.

Take heart, Jesus says. *There's more to the story.*

All will be well.

SURVIVOR

"For I know the plans I have for you," declares
the LORD, "plans to prosper you and not to harm
you, plans to give you hope and a future."

—JEREMIAH 29:11, NIV

I envy the stamina of people who volunteer for television's *Survivor*. Marooned in remote locales, shivering in the elements, competing in wacky challenges. Trying to "outwit, outplay, and outlast" and win a million bucks, if they're the sole survivor.

Then there's me, cancer survivor—plus seventeen million others, living through and beyond cancer.[17] Unlike television contestants, we didn't volunteer for this gig. None of us sent in videos or waved our arms and said to cancer, "Choose me!" There are great consolation prizes, though, like treasured moments with family. And mornings. And sunsets.

Like others, I've been sucked into a medical whirlwind. Faith is my lifeline, holding my feet to the ground. I'm using cream now for inflamed skin from a radiation burn. Those who have been through this say it will calm down. I hope so. Fatigue makes me feel like a road-weary warrior with thin emotional armor, but spring's early arrival this February fortifies me. A bit of sunshine does wonders.

Five to ten years of daily anti-hormone medicine is next on my plate. My doctor says this is the best way to prevent cancer's recurrence for those with hormone-receptor positive breast cancer cells, the kind that invaded my body. I had no idea what that phrase meant a year ago, floating in a bubble of good health far from the reality of the cancer that was secretly growing within me. He also says about 30 percent of women don't stay on this medicine. The side effects are too hard to live with, for many. What about me? Will I stick with it? I plan on it!

> *Joyce: You became a survivor at the moment of your diagnosis. I took the anti-hormone drug for nine and a half years. You can do this with God Almighty's hand holding you. I believe this!*

Over the last year, I've met people on rougher roads than mine. God doesn't cause cancer, but I believe God allows things into my (mostly cushy) life to mature me into the image of Jesus. I never grow when I'm not struggling. When I'm tempted to have a pity party, I need to stand on this boundless truth: "For our light and momentary troubles are achieving for us an eternal glory that far outweighs them all" (2 Cor. 4:17, NIV).

Unlike television rivals who connive to be the sole survivor, I'm encircled by people who wrap me in care, helping me outlast, outpray, and outwit cancer. The Word tells me life is about more than survival of the fittest. Jesus came for the lost, the last, the least. A sign I kept on my desk before I retired said, "Worry or Peace. You get to choose." I pray for inner calm when worry— fear's precursor—begins to worm its way into my brain. There's not enough space in my head for both.

Ash Wednesday marks the beginning of Lent, but for me every day is Easter. I'm a survivor.

With a future and a hope.

All will be well.

WONDERFUL LIFE

This is the day that the LORD has made;
let us rejoice and be glad in it.

—PSALM 118:24

Navigating cancer is like traveling in a foreign country. The language, people, and territory are strange. Anything that sounds familiar is welcome, like the bells that chime from my downtown church. Their music floats through the air, reaching my home a few miles away.

My neighbor discovered what church bells meant to her when she attended an intensive foreign language institute at a New England college. English was prohibited, but near her dorm a bell tower played hymns each day. She hummed along in her room as she studied. Soon she was living overseas, carrying music within to sustain her during long years in a lonely, unfamiliar place.

Church bells are traced back to Italy, where they called people to worship, to mourn the dead, to celebrate weddings, and to practice daily prayer. My daughter was in Assisi with a group of Presbyterians when a new pope was elected. Bells tolled the news from every church in town, waking her from a nap. Tara ran to a window and watched the happy scene below as people flooded into the streets to celebrate.

Bells have found their way into hospitals and cancer centers. Patients ring them when they reach a milestone. It's especially touching when it's a child. News reports show kids who have suffered through treatments ringing brass bells like it's Christmas morning and Santa just arrived.

About five hundred friends virtually celebrated with me on Facebook after I posted a picture yanking the brass bell at the local cancer center, Jim by my side. Not a soul commented on the peach fuzz that signaled my hair would someday return. Social media has its drawbacks, but the friends, support, and prayers I've gathered there have made this journey easier.

> **Art professor, her drawl audible:** Ring the bell of freedom! You're a warrior, Darlin'!
>
> **Oncology nurse:** The sound of that bell in my old clinic was like hearing angels sing!

The nurse's comment brought to mind our community theater's musical version of *It's a Wonderful Life* one snowy winter in the nineties. Jim and our two girls tried out and won singing roles. With twelve performances throughout December, it was a big commitment that required months of rehearsals. I was there, a theater mom, for every practice and show. Jimmy Stewart, our town's favorite son, starred as George Bailey in the 1947 film. Almost fifty years later, several original cast members were in our town for a weekend to honor the aging actor. Karolyn Grimes, who played Zuzu, clapped from the front row when our young Julie piped up, "Every time a bell rings, an angel gets its wings."[18]

During a snowstorm, a cast member couldn't get out of her icy lane, miles from town. She asked me to fill in, playing opposite Jim as George Bailey's mother. It was a packed house and I was nervous, but everyone helped me along. In real life, there's no rehearsal for cancer ahead of time, but like my family who memorized their parts for the show, lines of scripture are etched deep within me and rise to the surface when I need them most.

My relief in reaching this good place is tempered by prayers for others undergoing cancer treatments. But when one has a victory, it's a victory for all.

> **Cancer survivor:** *My burn scars from radiation remind me that God is always with me and has gotten me through many rough times.*
>
> **High school friend:** *Every time a bell rings, an angel is blessed!*

That brass bell's ring is the sweet sound of life. And I have a wonderful one.

All will be well.

VIGIL FIRES

When I called, you answered me;
you greatly emboldened me.
May all the kings of the earth praise you, LORD,
when they hear what you have decreed.

—PSALM 138:3-4, NIV

The last time we snuggled in bed before they left for New Zealand, I prayed the Three-in-One would protect my grandsons like they protected Saint Patrick. Then I told them stories I had gathered on my trip to the misty Emerald Isle. This is one, as I recall hearing it from our guide on the Hill of Tara, an ancient burial site where high kings were anointed to reign:

Patrick arrived on the shore of Ireland on Easter Eve, a sacred night for both Christians and pagan druids. No one was permitted to light a fire that night—under penalty of death—until the great fire of High King Legionnaire burned atop the Hill of Tara. (My Grandma Wesp first told me Ireland's renowned hill bears my daughter's name. Or is it the other way around?)

Patrick was no stranger to Ireland where he was once enslaved, yet many decades later he willingly returned. Captured as a teenage boy by pirates raiding Brittany's coast in the fifth century, he was brought to Ireland as a slave and for years herded sheep on lonely mountainsides, cold, hungry, and nearly naked. The God his parents told him about became real to him as he survived, alone in the elements. Patrick prayed a hundred times a day and as many times each night. Finally, God led him in a dream to escape and run to a ship about to sail. He came back many years later as a priest, after another dream in which he heard the Irish people cry out to God to send him to help them.

Not everyone was happy about his arrival. Patrick knew exactly what he was doing when he built a vigil bonfire on the beach. Druids, the king's advisers, looked across Ireland's gentle hills and were alarmed when they saw it. One of the wisest warned the king he must put out that fire or it would never die. He was right. Fires of faith still burn in Ireland, keeping vigil to the God Saint Patrick worshiped.[19]

My parents recalled an early era in aviation history when Dad flew into Penn State at night, before there was much of an airport. "I could hear the plane circling above, and I knew your dad was on it," Mother remembered. Daddy looked down and saw only darkness until finally somebody raced out and lit fires lining the landing strip. Little fires, glowing in the dark.

When I'm feeling lost, I welcome sparks of light to guide me home as well.

My hope is in the name of the Lord, who made the hills of Ireland, Pennsylvania, and New Zealand, where I had hoped to be with Tara's family right now. A nurse warned me the aftermath of thirty-six radiation treatments could drain my energy for months. I didn't want to hear it. Then visits to our kids in Ohio and Philly zonked me. I sighed and put away the folded clothes I'd piled on a bed for an adventure that was not to be. I ached to hold my grandchildren.

Psalm 138 powerfully describes God's faithfulness, and I look to it often. Many believers memorize psalms for strength in tough times. This psalm's eight verses can embolden you too.

A praying friend, Jean, understood and texted:

*God's arm and love stretch the whole way from
Pennsylvania to New Zealand and everywhere
in between. We can never be far from God, who
dwells with and within us.*

There's another story I told the boys about Patrick's men.
They tramped through enemy territory boldly singing the saint's
great prayer of protection, called a *lorica*, binding to themselves
the high name of the Trinity. It's said their adversaries saw only a
herd of deer, crying as they ran through the forest.[20]

"Is that really true?" Josiah, the eldest, asked doubtfully.

I smiled a grandma kind of smile. I've learned from Saint
Patrick that a song can carry me through the woods, all the way
to the other side. Perhaps a story can do that too. Do we sometimes ask the wrong questions? A verse from the Irish hymn we
know as "Be Thou My Vision" speaks my desire when I reach
the end of my days on earth:

> Great God of heaven, my victory won,
> may I reach heaven's joys, O bright heaven's Sun!
> Heart of my own heart, whatever befall,
> still be my vision, O Ruler of all. (UMH, no. 451)

All will be well.

The Practice of Celtic Prayer

All the earth bows down to you;
they sing praise to you,
they sing the praises of your name.

—PSALM 66:4, NIV

I began praying in the Celtic tradition while reading in preparation for my Celtic pilgrimage. Celtic Christianity is traced back to believers in the early centuries of the faith. According to Deborah K. Cronin in *Holy Ground: Celtic Christian Spirituality*, Saint Paul's letter to the Galatians was written to the Celts in Galatia.[21] Like early Hebrews, Celtic people lived close to the earth and depended upon God and their own resourcefulness for shelter, clothing, food, and warmth. Out of this intimate, earthy relationship arose the belief that creation is holy and life-giving. The number three was sacred before the arrival of Saint Patrick in Ireland; that devotion was easily transferred to the Sacred Three of Father, Son, and Spirit. A tale says he used a three-leaf clover to explain the Three-in-One.

The prayers of these people reflect the unwavering belief that humanity reflects God's image (see Genesis 1:27). Trust permeates Celtic prayers, often centered on mundane labor that composed their days, such as milking the cows, fishing the sea, and protecting families from harm.

"Be Thou My Vision" is an eighth-century Celtic hymn, writes Cronin. "Celtic Christians . . . most often surrounded by both water and the Divinity, sing the traditional words of this Celtic Christian hymn from the deep recesses of the heart."[22]

Many Celtic-style prayers offered today grew out of the spirit of the work of Alexander Carmichael, who tramped the hills of Scotland in the mid-1800s and early twentieth century. He paused at cottages and huts to record the prayers, folklore, ballads, and poetry of homemakers and farmers who depended on their faith to carry them through hardships, much like we who live with cancer do. Carmichael's life work was compiled into six volumes called *Carmina Gadelica,* which feature Christian and pre-Christian sayings.

Reading Celtic prayers inspired me to write this piece, entitled "Prayer for Hearth and Heart":

> I trust my embers to your care, O Sacred Three.
> May your angels guard them, Father.
> Tend their light this bitter night, sweet Spirit.
> Resurrect their flame with dawn's return, my
>   Jesus.

Why turn to this style of prayer now, when prayers are often spontaneous, unwritten, formless? I find it's comforting to connect with believers across the centuries. Their reverence for nature and sense of the immediacy of the Lord's presence strengthen my resolve to claim life is mine today.

* * *

Choose a natural setting that stirs praises to God. You can step outdoors, view creation through a window, or hold a rock or shell in your hands. Read a psalm or written prayer or create your own, praising God's hand for creating and sustaining this world.

Express thanks for the Sacred Three right there in the center of whatever turmoil your day may bring. Resources that aid this practice include *Christ Beside Me, Christ Within Me: Celtic Blessings* by Beth A. Richardson; *The Celtic Vision: Prayers, Blessings, Songs, and Invocations from the Gaelic Tradition* edited by Esther de Waal; *Celtic Daily Prayer: Prayers and Readings from the Northumbria Community*; and Marilyn Chandler McEntyre's *Christ, My Companion: Meditations on the Prayer of St. Patrick.*

WHAT POTTERS DO

O LORD, you are our Father;
we are the clay, and you are our potter;
we are all the work of your hand.

—ISAIAH 64:8

I watched Jim's hands at the potter's wheel, maneuvering mud as his foot pedaled away. He was bent over, intent on his creation. Again and again, he remolded his clay until satisfied with the final shape. He was my boyfriend back then, a biology major who spent more time in the pottery shop than in the bio lab. We still serve salads in the family-sized bowls he made.

I've never had Jim's knack for creating things with my hands, but I was intrigued by a Pittsburgh Theological Seminary class called "In God's Image: An Old Testament View of Dust and Clay." Yes, we would handle wet clay along with biblical stories, but how bad could that be?

As it turned out, pretty bad. My hands were too weak to manipulate clay, even on an electric wheel. After my mud ball flew off the wheel a few times, headed toward a good-natured neighbor, I decided I was safer hand-shaping an object that others kindly called an olive tray.

In contrast, consider the Master Potter, who "formed man from the dust of the ground, and breathed into his nostrils the breath of life; and the man became a living being" (Gen. 2:7). Did God get muddy making us, as potters do? We may think God had a mess on those holy hands, yet God took one look at this creation—made in the divine image—and declared, "Very good!"

As a cancer survivor, I've tried to see others through God's affirmation of original goodness. Saint Paul described us as "God's handiwork, created in Christ Jesus to do good works, which God prepared in advance for us to do" (Eph. 2:10, NIV). We're God's treasures, designed to spread God's goodness across the earth, beginning anew each morning wherever our feet hit the ground.

God placed Adam in a garden, surrounded by beauty and potential, with the chance to get dirt under his fingernails. He messed up royally and finger-pointed to Eve, who, according to the story, first fell into temptation. God, thank goodness, specializes in restoring order out of chaos—sometimes at great price. Our messes, failures, weaknesses, and even our diseases become steppingstones to fulfill a purpose greater than ourselves if we view them that way, trusting God and the scarred hands of Jesus to remold us again and again.

> Have thine own way, Lord! Have thine own way!
> Thou art the potter, I am the clay.
> Mold me and make me after thy will,
> while I am waiting, yielded and still. (UMH, no. 382)

In our pottery class we went in a workroom behind the seminary's Kelso Museum, where we handled shards of baked clay five and six thousand years old. I learned anew that mute objects convey hints of their past. Touching bits of pottery that prehistoric crafters—likely women—labored over gave me a sense of kinship with them, like I feel when I sip tea from one of Jim's mugs. Shattered pieces speak to the value of fragmented lives that seem beyond repair. The museum's pieced-together bowls and oil vessels tell stories of their creators; we too mirror sacred glimpses of God. Fracture lines allow light to shine through, revealing the commitment of those dedicated to reclaiming broken things.

> *Fellow student, Susan:* Your article brought
> back memories of things handed down to
> me. Remembering that although this vessel is
> cracked and wearing out, I am being renewed
> day by day.

I'm the Creator's restored vessel, fashioned from mud, bearing God's fingerprints, and more precious because of my scars.

All will be well.

THIS HOLY MYSTERY

"Do this, whenever you drink it,
in remembrance of me."

—1 CORINTHIANS 11:25, NIV

Communion Sundays came around four times a year when I was a kid, a pattern set by circuit-riding Methodist preachers on the American frontier in the 1700s. In the United Methodist denomination, Communion is considered a "holy mystery," which is an apt description of something beyond our comprehension. My parents felt that my twin sister and I were too young to understand the sacrament's meaning in grade school, so they sent us skipping out the church doors after Sunday school. We didn't bother telling them we climbed the tower of Old Main on our way across the Penn State campus toward home and paused to crawl over the smooth surface of the famous Nittany Lion. There was something else we never told them either. Kids are intuitive when it comes to things of the Spirit. We felt we were missing out on something sacred and decided to do something about it. One Sunday after we reached home, Marilyn grabbed a box of Ritz Crackers and I found a pitcher of juice in the fridge. We took our first Communion using what was familiar and within reach. We did it on our knees in our tiny bedroom closet, dresses and blouses shoved to the side, a safe place for a sacred secret.

Was it holy? Definitely. Was it mysterious? Of course. Was God present? Without a doubt.

Our folks were right; kids can't comprehend Communion. But who can? Jesus offers tangible symbols of himself, layered in the earthy substances of wheat and grapes, so we can enter into rituals with a childlike heart and soul, no matter who we are. If we come expectantly to the table, we find grace ingrained in the bread, pressed into the wine.

I look at the sacraments the way John Wesley, the founder of Methodism, explained them, as outward signs of an inward grace. Flimsy boundaries like gender and age can't box in grace, an extravagant expression of God's unlimited love. Tasting fresh bread and sipping fragrant wine nourish a sense of oneness with the Lord's physical body on earth—that is all of us in the body of Christ.

Pastor Kathy brought Communion to Jim and me on our shady breezeway one afternoon before my chemo sessions began. We pulled wicker chairs knee to knee, and then she prayed and anointed me in the name of the Sacred Three. Her visit prepared us spiritually for what I would go through physically with cancer treatments. I only took the sacrament once during my six months of chemo and missed it. (I was in isolation most of the time and could not be around other people.) Something happens to me when I take Communion that doesn't happen when I don't. It's part of the mystery.

Another mystery, the cross, is the most powerful signpost in my faith. The cross is a cruel form of torture and death, and it makes no more sense than an electric chair would dangling from a silver chain around my neck—until you know the blood-red love of Jesus poured out there. During Holy Week, a friend shared what Jesus said to his friends at their first Communion: "As the Father has loved me, so I have loved you; abide in my love" (John 15:9).

Communion is a come-as-you-are party, one I don't want to miss. Love is God's holy duct tape, holding me together and binding me to the Lord through others. I know so little about loving like Jesus but seek and pray for practical ways to show grace to others. God always provides, just as happened that morning when two little girls celebrated a Holy Mystery in their bedroom closet with crackers and orange juice.

In Jesus' name.

All will be well.

The Practice of Sacramental Living

Whatever you do, in word or deed, do
everything in the name of the Lord Jesus,
giving thanks to God the Father through him.

—COLOSSIANS 3:17

Living sacramentally includes every practice mentioned in this book and so much more. I've only skimmed the surface of the pleasures and challenges that accompany spiritual disciplines. This is awe-filled, attentive living, awake to the profound beauty and intense suffering that surround us.

Jesus used natural elements to convey spiritual truths, showing us our existence is both earth- and heaven-bound. Cancer has opened my eyes to the holy dimensions of every moment, to all things dedicated to bringing the fullness of God's love into the here and now. Sacramental living is living by the Great Commandment—loving God and loving our neighbors.

A bag of groceries from a food bank becomes holy when it feeds a hungry child. An eagle soaring overhead is holy when seen as part of God's creation to be protected, restored, and forever free. Picking up litter along a roadway is one of countless ways to respect God's command in Genesis to rule the earth honorably. People who knit, crochet, and quilt for others perform acts of sacred love, as do innumerable men and women who help lift the burdens of neighbors, near and far.

A person who chooses this lifestyle lays everything at the foot of the cross—desires, thoughts, actions, resources, attitudes, relationships, health, and past, present, and future—asking Jesus to transform their broken offering into something life-giving for others. It's surrendered living. It's non-judgmental living too, releasing as best we can people to God's care and forgiving from our depths anyone who caused us harm. The practice of sacramental living views life through a lens of love, even in an unkind, often ruthless world. Not sentimental, gushy love but sacrificial, unconditional agape love that welcomes family, friends, and strangers through the doors of our heart. Sacramental living recognizes and responds to that divine spark of God's Spirit in everyone.

* * *

We practice living sacramentally whenever our hands become the hands of Christ, encouraging or supporting someone else. How might you practice sacramental living? Think of a way you can serve your community. Ask your family members if they'd like to join you in a volunteer project. Do you have a hobby that might benefit others, such as baking or gardening? Are there ways in which you might curb your consumption or use fewer resources? Most of us have items in our home we no longer need, and these can be passed along to folks who could use them. Once you commit yourself to this way of life, chances are you'll discover you receive more than you give.

ALL DRESSED UP WITH SOMEPLACE TO GO

Clothe yourselves with the new self, created
according to the likeness of God in true
righteousness and holiness.

—EPHESIANS 4:24

My mom always made my sisters and me new dresses for Easter when we were children, carefully selecting cheerful fabrics from a vendor who brought samples to our home (this was before Jo-Ann Fabrics came to town). I still recall pressing my face into the sheer cotton dotted swiss, the choice one spring. Later, I sewed my own daughters' Easter finery when they were small.

The tradition of new clothing for Resurrection Day started as an outward sign of faith—new attire on the outside can reflect deeper things stirring inwardly. The early church required intense weeks of solemn preparations for converts to the faith. Finally, robed in white, they were baptized on Easter into new life in Jesus, putting on new selves, created to be pleasing and holy to the Lord.

During Holy Week, Tara messaged from New Zealand:

*Eli's church schoolteacher mentioned he spent
most of the hour just hanging out in their
makeshift tomb.*

Something, perhaps a sacred sense of mystery, attracted my young grandson to that closed-in space, much like my sister and I huddled in our tiny closet for our version of Communion. Mary Magdalene hung around the tomb too. Feet wet with dew and eyes swollen from tears, she was the first follower to encounter the risen Christ.

Glad to see her and eager to comfort her, Jesus called out, "Mary!" Jesus said her name and changed her world. She looked up and answered, "Rabbouni!" (See John 20:11-16.)

Mary's beloved rabbi and teacher was fully alive. Jesus' first recorded words, stepping out of death from a dark tomb, were to a woman who wondered how she could ever live without him. In that single word, he spoke life into Mary's heart and then sent her to tell the others. Her feet now flying, Mary was the first person to share the Good News—an apostle to the Apostles.

Sweet Jesus, how incautiously you love us! You break down walls, call us by name, and restore relationships. The Christian life is measured by an old rugged cross—before and after. We live by grace on the better side of Easter, following the Giver of new beginnings.

I'm thankful to the One who knows every (new) hair on my head. I'm happy not to show off any selections from my bonnet collection this Easter. I think I'll dress in white, though, for new life. The report of my first diagnostic mammogram says things look normal. New possibilities are unfolding on the better side of cancer, including a new name for my weekly newspaper column. I'm no longer texting through cancer, praise God; I'm a survivor who is "Texting Thru Recovery."

This was a year of uncertainty and wonder. Though gray-haired and scarred, inside I'm stronger and more intact because of my cancer journey, more convinced of God's unwavering faithfulness. And certainly richer for friendships and wisdom gained along the way.

> **Sue:** *You're wrapped in the loving arms of our great God. It will take time to feel your energetic self, but it certainly is around the corner. Be patient with yourself. Everything you know will be richer and more meaningful, and you will take nothing for granted. People have come into your life who wouldn't have otherwise. You've learned to rely on others more. You're touched by God to continue God's work in the same and different ways. You're in my constant prayers. Your life will never be the same again, but better.*

Trusting my tomorrows to Jesus, who knows my name, and yours. A beginning, not an end.

All will be well.

ALL WILL BE WELL,
AND ALL WILL BE WELL

Be brave and strong! ... The LORD your God
will always be at your side, and he will
never abandon you.

—DEUTERONOMY 31:6, CEV

Finally. My book proposal was in the mail. Would it be accepted by the first publisher I approached with my story? Would I become the Grandma Moses of writers, beginning my career as a book author after age seventy? With my blog underway and my newspaper column receiving positive comments, I felt like I was doing what God created me to do. I'd accomplished a few things on my bucket list, and my grandchildren were moving back to the States from New Zealand. To Pittsburgh, sixty miles from us, thank God!

And then, this.

Cancer survivors know a remote shadow may be hiding somewhere, waiting to change the course of our lives again. A distant possibility, easy to brush aside until we have reason to think differently. I'd had a constant ache like a stubborn urinary tract infection that wouldn't go away. That was the first sign something wasn't right. My doctor ordered a CT scan. I opened the report on the hospital portal two days later and suddenly understood why I was so miserable. A tumor—or tumors—had fractured my sacrum (part of the pelvis). Other lesions were scattered about as well, too much data for my brain to absorb.

When I approached Jim that night, he immediately read my pale face, switched off the television, and sat beside me. We read each word of the report in dry-mouth disbelief. "This can't be happening!" he groaned. I felt woozy, like I'd been hit in the head with a bowling ball. I'm infinitely glad we received this news in the privacy of each other's arms—we didn't have to disguise our anguish.

We know little about navigating a second journey through cancer, but we know this: Prayers carried us when I was first diagnosed with breast cancer, and we covet them again.

All will be well.

* * *

It's 5 a.m., and I'm sitting in my fluffy white robe at the kitchen table. A burning vanilla candle, a cup of tea, and a circling bat, zooming up and down the stairwell (yes, you read that right) are my companions.

Hours earlier, before I opened that report, my hairdresser, Brenda, invited Jim and me to her church for a healing service. She knew I was hurting, but not about this report. I had to do something. To take control. To battle this nightmare. Within an hour of my world crumbling for a second time, folks surrounded Jim and me, bathing us in prayer.

Afterward, I needed the comfort of familiar arms. Jim and I sat with my mentor and friend, Sue, who shared from her deep well of strength as a retired nurse who worked with women living with breast cancer. "There is hope," she said. "You will live. Jesus is with you, above you, below you, beside you." Her affirmation echoed the prayer of Saint Patrick, Ireland's patron saint. God is everywhere. There is nowhere God is not.

All will be well.

The hard part, what hurts my heart, is sharing this bad report with my family. I love them so. Jesus knows this. I must trust them to him, and they must trust me to him as well.

Strangely, my joy in living intensifies, like the way stars grow brighter in the dark. On Monday, Pastor Denny stopped by and anointed me for healing. I've been smeared with the oil of God's Spirit. I don't understand it, but I want it.

Messages like this from longtime friend Pastor Eric Park flooded in, after I posted my news:

> Hi Jan. I just read your most recent blog post. I
> have no words, friend, just a heart full of love,
> tears that commingle with yours, and a faith
> that connects us deeply. As you enter into a
> new segment of the journey and a new fight,
> know that we are praying for you, Jim, and your
> family in a "without ceasing" kind of urgency.
> Thank you for allowing us to stand with you
> upon the sacred ground of your struggle. And
> thank you for all the ways that you remind
> me that not even a cancer diagnosis takes
> us beyond the realm of what God can heal,
> redeem, and restore. You are not alone in this,
> friend. And you are loved.

All will be well.

***

In the fourteenth century, Julian of Norwich described Jesus coming to her in a divine revelation of love. She fell deathly ill at thirty. Her priest came to minister the last rites and told Julian to fix her eyes on Christ, suffering on the cross. As she did, she was healed. She is best remembered for these words that she received from Christ during her divine revelation: "All shall be well, and all shall be well, and all manner of thing shall be well." Words born out of suffering speak truth into mine. A shattering of bone brings an unwelcome chapter to my own story I had hoped never to write. I know it ends in the enveloping love of God, but I don't know the path that leads me there.

All will be well.

With all my prayers, one thing I didn't pray about was that darn bat. It's a confused, frightened creature flying in the dark, much like me. To some Native Americans, bats symbolize death and rebirth because they sleep in the belly of the earth and are reborn every night.[23] I released an unholy holler when this one circled me in the stairwell; a sliver of my own agony was expelled in that scream. With a calming sip of tea, I came to see this poor thing as a winged messenger telling me that, yes, I will die some-day and be reborn into the fullness of God's presence.

But not yet.

When I led activities at a retirement community, it was an honor for my staff and me to help residents live well. As their end drew near, it was an equal honor to help them die well.

I have more living to do, friends. Please pray I do it with grace.

All will be well.

GOODBYE, POPCORN

God loved the people of this world so much that he
gave his only Son, so that everyone who has faith
in him will have eternal life and never really die.

—JOHN 3:16, CEV

God is with us, and all will be well. I didn't doubt when I signed
up for hospice care that it was the right thing to do. These are
caring, compassionate people whose total goal is my comfort. We
can never know how much time we have, but as I've said before,
I trust myself to the hands of God. As Victor Raymond Edman
reminds us in *The Disciplines of Life*, "Never doubt in the dark
what God told you in the light."[24]

I regret that I won't see my book, *Texting Through Cancer: Ordinary Moments of Community, Love, and Healing*, be published by
Upper Room Books in March 2021. It is an example of letting go
and letting God handle all the details, like trusting my publisher
and Amazon to help distribute it. All of life, in the end, is about
letting go to the Great I AM.

I'm incredibly grateful to the *Indiana Gazette* for these four
years to share my journey through cancer, which is now nearing
its end. I've been blessed by hundreds of you, my readers. No one
hoped it would come to this, but all stories reach a conclusion.
I'm confident that angels will escort me when my time comes.

The other night I awoke as Jim was making popcorn downstairs. I smelled buttery memories collected over our fifty years together. I wave and say, "Goodbye, popcorn!" lightheartedly. God is teaching me to detach bit by bit from treasures of the past. While memories and people are wrapped in love, detachment says there is a time and place for everything to say goodbye until we are finally immersed in the Love of all Love.

A friend told me that many people will mourn as I leave that final shore. Sadly, I turn to board my boat. That's when I see a crowd of folks on the other side, waving me home. Jesus is rowing my boat, caring for me as he always has and will do into eternity. O Lord, I don't grasp what that means except to know my loving Lord presses me close.

Perfect love casts out fear, my friends.

"Jesus loves me! This I know, for the Bible tells me so" (UMH, no. 191).

All will be well.

A WORD OF THANKS

I stood at the Wailing Wall in Jerusalem and pulled little scraps of paper from my coat pocket. In tiny handwriting, they contained names of everyone I remembered in prayer. I crammed them into crevices and backed away, the proper way to respect that holy spot. I feel like I'm doing the same here, trying to honor everyone who in this case has prayed and loved me throughout cancer. It's probably not what many authors would do, but I'm me, living with a disease that makes this the time and place to thank people for standing with me.

This book is before you because people pushed me to write it, among them author Natalie Glaser and friend Henry "Hank" Clawson, who bugged me to complete it. Thank you! My twin sister and loving friend, Marilyn Watrous Emanuel, helped me write with clarity and edited for me. She is a prayer warrior, like most everyone mentioned here. Kim Young edited the first draft I sent off and was part of my first Christian writers fellowship. I'm grateful for practical encouragers who believed in me as a writer, especially Linda Strawcutter, Jean Rickard, and my treasured Wednesday morning study gang.

Indiana Gazette editor Jason Levan took a chance when I suggested writing a column, which I submitted weekly to religion page editor, Heather Blake. Thanks to all the *Gazette* family.

Friends have cried and laughed with me. Faye Catlos and Sue Majoris, thank you beyond words for being there when life unraveled. In addition to my twin sister, my other siblings, Carol Naspinsky and George Watrous, continually lifted me in prayer and were only a phone call away. Some have traveled with me in other ways. Tina Whitehead was my roommate to the Holy Lands. Judy Shipley was my roomie on my Celtic pilgrimage, and Rebecca Cole-Turner was an insightful guide turned friend. These life-changing journeys expanded my vision of the great heart of God.

Hundreds of Facebook friends and *Gazette* readers have prayed for me and sent messages that inspired this book. Your encouragement keeps me writing, week after week. Dr. Roger Owens of Pittsburgh Theological Seminary read sample entries and suggested I submit them to Upper Room Books, where I first worked with acquisitions editor Joanna Bradley Kennedy.

To the people who have sustained me, be assured your names are tucked in a corner of my heart. God knows who you are and every stitch of love and prayer that hems our stories together. Standing with me are Elizabeth and Raphael from Kenya and my fantastic writing circle; St. Thomas More centering prayer friends; Saturday morning prayer fellowship; the hilarious CRS book club; Jim's master gardening buddies; everyone who sent texts, cards, messages, food, and gifts; my wonderful activities staffers at St. Andrew's Village; the Operation Sunday School team; my extended family and nieces and nephews; supportive fellow warriors in COURAGE and Cancer*, Indiana Regional Medical Center (IRMC) breast cancer group, and Joyce Landacre; State College Area High School, Indiana University of Pennsylvania, and Pittsburgh Theological Seminary spiritual formation classmates; our neighbors; Sisters & Sanity friends; Pastor Kathy's Wednesday afternoon group; church prayer team

---

* Following the author's diagnosis of advanced cancer, Jan joined with like-minded friends to begin a monthly support group, COURAGE and Cancer, for anyone who lives with cancer. Visit @courageandcancer on Facebook.

members; Methodist Youth Fellowship kids I led in the past who have amazingly remained in touch; our pastors; everyone at Grace United Methodist Church; and Young Life leaders who made Jesus real to me.

Thanks to Casting for Recovery of Western Pennsylvania for a fantastic fly-fishing experience; to folks of First Presbyterian Church of Pasadena, Pasadena, Texas; Epworth United Methodist Church, Rehoboth Beach, Delaware; and St. Thomas More Roman Catholic Church in Indiana, Pennsylvania; and, of course, Hamburg United Methodist Church outside Buffalo, New York. I feel the warmth of the quilt, shawls, and prayers from all of you.

My oncologists, Dr. Gopala Ramenini and Dr. Adam Brufsky, and their staffs at IRMC, the Hillman Cancer Center, and Magee Women's Hospital, have given me more time to love and write. To a corps of cancer survivors and those sweet souls who have passed into eternity, thank you for leading the way for me and others.

To Jim, thank you for our lifetime together. You've put up with my writing daily for decades, surrounded by piles of papers and books. You were the first to tell me I could be a professional writer and author, and you edited my work. You keep me laughing, even as we sometimes mourn together; your love and care are unwavering on this unpredictable road rally. I'll love you forever.

Our beloved children, Brett, Tara, and Julie, and our grandchildren, are my best reasons to keep on fighting. Josiah and Eli, who are found in the pages of this book, and the Kalu kids— Fiona, Melody, and Josiah—are written on the grandma page of my heart. You are always in my prayers.

I have an inner assurance that this is only the beginning of an unending journey with the Sacred Three, to whom I owe everything. On this side of eternity and the next, all will be well.

ABOUT THE AUTHOR

Janet Watrous Woodard, 1948–2020

Jan grew up in State College, Pennsylvania, the child of a university professor father and an English teacher mother. Following her 1969 marriage, she lived in the small college town of Indiana, Pennsylvania, where she and her husband raised three children. She, her family, and her town celebrated *It's a Wonderful Life*, the film starring the town's favorite son, Jimmy Stewart. Although hers was no romanticized story, she loved Indiana, and her positive attitude toward life reflected her deep faith.

Jan believed in the transformative power of words and she was a writer from an early age. She was editor in chief of her high school newspaper and later was an award-winning journalist who wrote countless newspaper and magazine articles. For ten years she was a roving writer for her denomination, The United Methodist Church.

Jan not only told her own story but also helped others tell theirs. She led and facilitated retreats, workshops, classes, and writing groups. A lifelong leader and learner, Jan returned to school at age sixty to complete a master's degree in adult and community education. She then relished serving residents as the activity coordinator at a senior living facility.

Three years after her retirement, when Jan discovered her tumor, her husband Jim said the very first thing she wanted to do was to use it for good. So she started transparently telling her story, week by week. Her column, "Texting Thru Cancer," later became "Texting Thru Recovery," and was published both in *The Indiana Gazette* and her blog, janwoodard.com. Inspired by Julian of Norwich (the first woman to publish a book in English), Jan closed each of her posts with the words "All will be well." In the four-year run of her column, she never missed a submission, despite periods of debilitating illness.

Jan used words to teach and heal. With extraordinary courage and vulnerability, she shared her journey, and her words were a balm to this aching world. Jan didn't just tell her story; she lived it. She insisted a life well lived is one in which you look outside yourself and toward the needs of others. She did this her entire life.

Through her pilgrimage to the Iona Abbey of Scotland and classes in spiritual formation at Pittsburgh Theological Seminary, Jan's faith was nourished and deepened. Her study of Celtic Christian spirituality provided an ancient language of faith that grounded her in a fresh way. She practiced gratitude for simple, everyday things, believing all of it was a gift.

From the beginning of her battle with breast cancer, Jan's goal was to be truthful about her own experience and to use it to inspire and comfort others. Jan was not fond of trite clichés or false comforts. She bravely confronted the truth that everything would not end happily ever after. Still, she had hope. Though she would miss those she leaves behind, she insisted she was not afraid of death. She knew there was more that lies beyond this earthly life.

Jan's final years were transformative because she chose to make her most private battle public and made a heart commitment to pen her words for Jesus. Her family hopes this book continues her legacy of hopeful, helpful compassion, so others may pass this along.

Early on the morning of Wednesday, June 3, 2020, surrounded by her husband and family, Janet Watrous Woodard transitioned from this life to the next. She described her destination as a final shore where she would be finally immersed in the Love of all Love. Now Jan is safely on the other side of that shore, embraced in the arms of her Savior, still reminding us that—come what may—all will be well.

Jan's dream to publish a book is realized with the publication of *Texting Through Cancer: Ordinary Moments of Community, Love, and Healing.* Her family is grateful to *The Indiana Gazette* for printing her column and to Upper Room Books for publishing her book, especially editorial director Joanna Bradley Kennedy and freelance editor Amy Lyles Wilson. Amy worked closely and compassionately with Jim Woodard and Marilyn Watrous Emanuel to prepare Jan's manuscript for publication.

NOTES

1. Veronica Mary Rolf, *Julian of Norwich* (Downers Grove, IL: IVP Academic, 2018), 148.
2. Marilyn Chandler McEntyre, *Christ, My Companion: Meditations on the Prayer of St. Patrick* (Grand Rapids, MI: Baker Books, 2008), 40.
3. McEntyre, *Christ, My Companion*, 47.
4. Margery Williams, *The Velveteen Rabbit*. (New York: Hyperion, 1977), 4.
5. Shelley Taylor et al., "Biobehavioral responses to stress in females: tend-and-befriend, not fight-or-flight," https://www.ncbi.nlm.nih.gov/pubmed/10941275, accessed December 10, 2019.
6. W. Phillip Keller. *A Shepherd Looks at Psalm 23* (Grand Rapids, MI: Zondervan, 2008), 56.
7. John Donne, *No Man Is an Island,* originally published in *Devotions Upon Emergent Occasions* (1624).
8. St. Peter's Episcopal Church, Lewes, Delaware, email correspondence with author, December 6, 2019.
9. William Herbert Carruth, *Each in His Own Tongue and Other Poems* (New York: Putnam's Sons, 1909), http://www.theotherpages.org/poems/carruth1.html, accessed December 13, 2019.
10. Gus Hahn, "My Buddy" (New York: Remick Music Corporation, 1922), https://commons.wikimedia.org/wiki/File:My_Buddy.pdf, accessed January 12, 2020.
11. *The Spiritual Formation Bible: Growing in Intimacy with God through Scripture* (Grand Rapids, MI: Zondervan, 1999), 1076.
12. Phillips Brooks, "O Little Town of Bethlehem" (1868), https://www.umcdiscipleship.org/resources/history-of-hymns-o-little-town-of-bethlehem, accessed December 20, 2019.
13. C. Michael Hawn, https://www.umcdiscipleship.org/resources/history-of-hymns-o-little-town-of-bethlehem.
14. Brooks, "O Little Town of Bethlehem."

15. Fiona Kalu, *Your Journey: 40 Days to Reflect on Your Walk with the Lord*, https://www.amazon.com/Your-Journey-Days-Reflect-Walk-ebook /dp/B01BA0EE2S.

16. https://www.ourcatholicprayers.com/st-patricks-breastplate.html.

17. American Cancer Society https://www.cancer.org/latest-news /population-of-us-cancer-survivors-grows-to-nearly-17-million .html, accessed by editor on August 5, 2020.

18. *Wonderful Life*, the musical by Shelton Harnick, performed by the Indiana Players, is based on the movie *It's a Wonderful Life*.

19. https://www.irish-genealogy-toolkit.com/legend-of-saint-patrick .html.

20. Commonly attributed to St. Patrick as his *lorica* (prayer of protection). Available online as "Irish Prayer," https://www.catholic.org /prayers/prayer.php?p=3290, accessed March 9, 2019. This is commonly called "The Prayer of St. Patrick" or "The Deer's Cry," as well as "St. Patrick's Breastplate." My favorite rendition, arranged by Shaun Davey and sung by Rita Connolly, can be found on You-Tube: "The Deer's Cry, Rita Connolly Sings at Powerscourt."

21. Deborah K. Cronin, *Holy Ground* (Nashville, TN: Upper Room Books, 1999), 33.

22. Cronin, *Holy Ground*, 18.

23. http://www.pure-spirit.com/more-animal-symbolism/222-pure -spirit-minneapolis-st-paul-dog-training-and-international-all -species-animal-communication-bat, accessed January 12, 2020.

24. Victor Raymond Edman, *The Disciplines of Life* (Minneapolis, MN: World Wide Publications 1948), 33, https://archive.org/details /disciplinesoflif00edma, accessed by editor September 23, 2020.